OSCEs IN
PAEDIATRICS

For Churchill Livingstone

Publisher Timothy Horne
Project Editor Jane Shanks
Project Controller Frances Affleck
Design Direction Erik Bigland

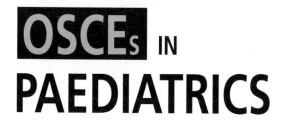

OSCEs IN PAEDIATRICS

A KHAN MBChB BMSc MRCP MRCPCH

Specialist Registrar in Paediatric Respiratory Medicine
The Hospital for Sick Children
Great Ormond Street
London, UK

H PANDYA MBChB MRCP MRCPCH

Lecturer in Paediatrics, Department of Paediatrics,
Leicester Royal Infirmary, Leicester

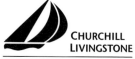

CHURCHILL
LIVINGSTONE

EDINBURGH LONDON NEW YORK PHILADELPHIA SYDNEY
TORONTO 1999

CHURCHILL LIVINGSTONE
An imprint of Harcourt Brace & Company Limited

Robert Stevenson House, 1–3 Baxter's Place, Leith Walk, Edinburgh EH1 3AF, UK

First published 1999

ISBN 0 443 05728 1

British Library Cataloguing in Publication Data
A catalogue record for this book is available from the British Library.

Library of Congress Cataloging in Publication Data
A catalog record for this book is available from the Library of Congress.

Medical knowledge is constantly changing. As information becomes available, changes in treatment, procedures, equipment and the use of drugs become necessary. The authors and publishers have, as far as it is possible, taken care to ensure that the information given in the text is accurate and up to date. However, readers are strongly advised to confirm that the information, especially with regard to drug usage, complies with current legislation and standards of practice.

The
publisher's
policy is to use
**paper manufactured
from sustainable forests**

Printed in China
GCC/01

FOREWORD

The last few years have seen the publication of a number of excellent textbooks of paediatrics, designed to provide the clinical medical student with the core information needed to pass the final clinical examination and to form the basis for further postgraduate education in paediatrics. Meanwhile, the examination process in many universities has seen the displacement of the long and short case evaluation by the Objective Structured Clinical Examination (OSCE). Although generally welcomed by both candidates and examiners alike, as providing a fairer and broader test of the student clinical skills, the introduction of the OSCE has generated considerable anxiety. This book will do much to allay these anxieties and is likely to prove popular for some years to come.

Its main strength is, however, that it provides an excellent teaching and revision resource which will be attractive to many starting higher qualification. The authors have ensured that by including over 100 topics in 5 separate OSCE examinations, all the major areas of paediatrics have been covered using a Question and Answer approach.

Professor A. D. Milner
1998

ACKNOWLEDGEMENTS

We are grateful to Dr C. Stern, Mr H. Ward, Professor A. D. Milner and the departments of paediatrics, medical illustration and cytogenetics of Guy's and St Thomas' Hospital and King's College Hospital, London, for providing the material for this book. Dr R. Thwaites' contribution of carefully reading the entire manuscript and providing constructive critical comments has also been particularly invaluable.

ABBREVIATIONS

Units of measurement are given in parentheses when appropriate.

ABG	Arterial blood gases
ALL	Acute lymphoblastic leukaemia
ASD	Atrial septal defect
ASOT	Anti-streptolysin titre
BE	Base excess
BP	Blood pressure
CF	Cystic fibrosis
Cl	Chloride (mmol/L)
CMV	Cytomegalovirus
CPK	Creatinine phosphokinase
CSF	Cerebrospinal fluid
CRP	C-reactive protein
CT	Computed tomography
CXR	Chest X-ray
DIOS	Distal intestinal obstruction syndrome
DMD	Duchenne muscular dystrophy
DMSA	Dimercaptic succinic acid
DTPA	Diethyltriamine pentaacetic acid
ECG	Electrocardiography
EEG	Electroencephalography
EFA	Essential fatty acids
ESR	Erythrocyte sedimentation rate
FBC	Full blood count
GFR	Glomerular filtration rate
G6PD	Glucose-6-phosphate dehydrogenase
Hb	Haemoglobin (g/dL)
HCO_3	Bicarbonate (mmol/L)
HS	Hereditary spherocytosis
ITP	Idiopathic thrombocytopenic purpura
IVU	Intravenous urography
JVP	Jugular venous pressure
K	Potassium (mmol/L)
LP	Lumbar puncture
M,C&S	Microscopy, culture and sensitivity
MCUG	Micturating cystourethrogram

MDI	Metered dose inhaler
MMR	Measles, Mumps, Rubella
Na	Sodium (mmol/L)
NAI	Non-accidental injury
NEC	Necrotizing enterocolitis
P_{CO_2}	Partial pressure of carbon dioxide (kPa)
PDA	Patent ductus arteriosus
PEFR	Peak expiratory flow rate
Plat	Platelets ($\times 10^9$/L)
P_{O_2}	Partial pressure of oxygen (kPa)
RBC	Red blood cells
REM	Rapid eye movement
SSPE	Subacute sclerosing panencephalitis
SVT	Supraventricular tachycardia
TLE	Temporal lobe epilepsy
U	Urea (mmol/L)
U&E	Urea + electrolytes
URTI	Upper respiratory tract infection
US	Ultrasound
UTI	Urinary tract infection
VSD	Ventricular septal defect
WCC	White cell count ($\times 10^9$/L)

CONTENTS

INTRODUCTION

This book is written with the dual aim of providing medical students with an idea of what is involved in the objectively structured clinical examination (OSCE) in paediatrics as well as teaching paediatrics. As a form of assessment it is gradually replacing the short case long case plus viva which has been traditionally used in the UK. The cases used in the examination are, in general, practically oriented and, most importantly, the objectivity in the marking is emphasized – hence the title. It consists predominantly of systems examination, pictures of clinical signs, radiological investigations, data interpretation, history taking and 'what would you do now' type scenarios. The areas covered relate largely to primary and secondary care paediatrics; the occasional question in this book touches on tertiary practice. Some questions are therefore deliberately difficult and could easily have been included in an MRCP examination!

Basic sciences were considered important areas to be taught and tested when the latest national undergraduate curriculum changes were introduced – we have therefore incorporated these areas into the questions and tried to adhere to those situations where theory has a direct relevance to practice.

A whole chapter in this book has been written exclusively to cover the five most used systems examinations in the OSCE. The chapter is deliberately brief with the intention to remind rather than teach de novo and to give an idea of how marks are allocated.

We have tried to keep the questions up to date and hope that students find them stimulating. We also hope that examiners/medical educationalists who set final paediatric examinations may find some of the material used here useful in setting their own assessments.

Finally, we would welcome any comments or criticisms from readers of this book.

A. Khan
H. Pandya

CLINICAL EXAMINATION OF SYSTEMS

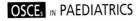

Checklist for examination of the cardiovascular system

Inspection	*Dysmorphic features*	Down and Turner syndrome
	Cyanosis and pallor	
	Respiratory rate	
	Clubbing	Cyanotic heart disease, e.g. Fallot's tetralogy
	Jugular venous pressure (JVP)	Usually unnecessary in children
	Scars	Look front and back Central sternotomy – open heart surgery, e.g. atrial septal defect (ASD) and ventricular septal defect (VSD) Left thoracotomy – pulmonary artery banding or patent ductus arteriosus (PDA) closure
Palpation		Pulse rate, rhythm, character (water-hammer of aortic regurgitation or bounding of PDA) and volume of radial pulse. Check for radio-femoral delay
	Apex beat	May be visible. Measure down from the sternal angle and the 2nd left intercostal space. If palpation is uncertain check right side to exclude dextrocardia
	Thrill	Use palm of hand or fingers. Check for thrill in the suprasternal notch for aortic stenosis. Presence of thrill indicates a murmur of at least grade 4/6
	Parasternal heave	
	Liver	Look for in all children

Auscultation

Heart sounds	2nd heart sound is loud when pulmonary blood flow is increased, e.g. ASD and VSD, or when pulmonary hypertension is present Presence of splitting should be mentioned if heard. To discriminate between the different causes of this is not expected at the undergraduate level Ejection click – if early, indicates aortic or pulmonary valve stenosis
Murmurs	Description should include: grade (1–6), loudest area, radiation, timing (systolic, diastolic) and duration (e.g systolic or pansystolic) Posture – assess the murmur in different postures. Lying down (venous hum disappears), sitting up (pulmonary flow murmurs decrease) or rolling the patient over to the left side (accentuates mitral valve-related murmurs). Listen to back – PDA, pulmonary stenosis and coarctation of aorta

Blood pressure Always offer to measure this; usually, this will not be required

Checklist for examination of the respiratory system

Inspection	*Cyanosis*	Ask to look at lips
	Respiratory distress	Suprasternal, intercostal or subcostal recession
	Noises	Audible stridor or wheeze. A child is stredulous if the inspiratory noises are thought to emanate from the neck. Stertorous inspiratory noises emanate from the nasopharyngeal area
	Chest deformity	Pectus excavatum (depressed sternum – usually idiopathic), pectus carinatum (prominent chest – asthma or other chronic obstructive condition) or asymmetry Harrison's sulci – retracted costal cartilages, indicate chronic respiratory conditions, e.g. asthma
	Respiratory rate	Count over 10–15 s. Be precise in answer
	Clubbing	Consider cystic fibrosis or bronchiectasis
Palpation	*Tracheal deviation*	Feel gently in the suprasternal notch
	Apex beat	
	Chest expansion	
	Vocal fremitus	
Percussion		*Warn* child that you are going to tap the chest. Compare both sides of the chest. Locate the upper border of the liver. Remember to percuss the back
	Note – most aspects of palpation and percussion are not required in the examination of an infant	
Auscultation	*Air entry*	Is it symmetrical, absent or reduced

	Breath sounds	Vesicular (normal) or bronchial (associated with consolidation or collapse)
	Added sounds	Conducted upper airway sounds Wheezes – usually in expiration only Crepitations – fine, e.g. pulmonary oedema or coarse as in bronchiectasis or chronic lung disease
	Whispering pectoriloquy – if bronchial breathing is suspected	

Checklist for examination of the cranial nerves

1. Olfactory nerve	Rarely tested	Should however, be offered for examination
2. Optic nerve	Visual acuity	>3 years – use stycar matching letters >5 years – use Snellen charts
	Visual fields	Use confrontation perimetry. Central scotomas are rare in children. Look for homonymous hemianopia (secondary to cerebral haemorrhage) or bitemporal hemianopia (secondary to craniopharyngioma)
	Fundoscopy	Should be offered for examination. Usually will be asked to perform separately if there is pathology present and the pupils will have been dilated. Look for papilloedema, retinal pigmentation and optic atrophy
3, 4 and 6: **Oculomotor nerve** **Trochlear nerve** **Abducens nerve**		Tested by checking external ocular movements. 3rd nerve palsy causes pupil dilatation with absent light reflexes, ptosis and deviation of the eye downwards and out. 4th nerve palsy results in the

		eye being unable to be abducted while looking down. 6th nerve palsy results in a convergent squint and failure of abduction
5. Trigeminal nerve	*Motor*	Ask child to open mouth against resistance
	Sensory	Ophthalmic, maxillary and mandibular divisions must be checked
7. Facial nerve	*Motor*	Ask child to screw eyes shut, raise eyebrows, blow cheeks and smile. Lower motor neurone lesion causes ipsilateral weakness
	Sensory	7th nerve supplies sensation to anterior two-thirds of tongue – rarely requires to be tested. Corneal reflex should not be tested in the conscious child
8. Vestibulocochlear nerve		Deafness, if present, should be differentiated into sensorineural or conductive by using Weber's and Rinne's tests
9 and 10. Glossopharyngeal vagus nerve		Ask child to say 'ah' and look for palatal movement. Affected nerve side does not elevate. Dysarthria, difficulty in speech and swallowing may be present
11. Spinal accessory nerve		Ask child to shrug shoulders. Turn head to side against resistance
12. Hypoglossal nerve		Look for tongue fasciculation – a sign of lower motor neurone lesion. Upon tongue protrusion unilateral nerve lesion will cause deviation to side of lesion

Checklist for examination of the gastrointestinal system

General assessment

Hands	*Clubbing*	Cystic fibrosis, inflammatory bowel disease
	Pallor	
	Koilonychia	Iron deficiency
	Palmar erythema	Liver failure
Face	*Jaundice*	
	Periorbital oedema	
	Spider naevi	
	Mouth	Ulcers of Crohn's disease
Inspection of abdomen	*Scars*	Check renal angle
	Distension	
	Masses	
	Hernias	Ask patient to cough and observe for this. Umbilical hernias are common in healthy Afrocaribbean infants
	Hydroceles	

Palpation		Ask the child first if the abdomen hurts *While observing the child's face* superficially palpate the whole abdomen. Continue deep palpation of whole abdomen
	Liver edge	Start from right iliac fossa
	Spleen	Start from right iliac fossa – splint the lower rib cage posteriorly with left hand. To exclude smaller splenic enlargement turn the child half onto his right side and palpate again
	Kidneys	Bimanual examination
	Ascites	Shifting dullness and fluid thrill. Examine for this only if there is: evidence of liver failure, abdominal distension, hepatomegaly or oedema

Percussion	*Liver*	Percuss upper border to exclude hyperinflation causing

		apparent hepatomegaly. Measure size of enlarged organs with ruler
	Spleen	
Auscultation	*Renal bruit*	
	Bowel sounds	
Anus and rectum		*Offer only*, to examine this. You will not be expected to do this in the examination

Checklist for a motor neurological examination of the legs

Inspection	*Posture*	'Frog's legs' posture is usually indicative of hypotonia. Opisthotonic posturing is found in conditions leading to hypertonia
	Fasciculation	
	Muscle bulk	Wasting occurs in cerebral palsy. Calf hypertrophy in Duchenne muscular dystrophy
	Asymmetry	
	Scars	May provide evidence of tendon repair
	Lower back	Look for spinal abnormalities, e.g. spinal dysraphism
Gait		Ask patient to walk in a straight line. Increase difficulty by trying toe to heel walking and hopping. Look for ataxia, wide-based gait (cerebellar ataxia), hemiplegic gait, tip-toe walking, etc.
Rising from supine		Look specifically for Gower's sign

Tone	Remember to look for ankle clonus (more than three beats is sustained clonus) and range of movement
Power	Assess grade of power: Grade 0 – No movement 1 – Flicker of movement 2 – Antigravity movement 3 – Fair 4 – Below normal strength 5 – Normal
Reflexes	Try reinforcing the reflexes before concluding that they might be absent. Plantar reflex is often equivocal in children. It must be done however, as it may provide evidence of pyramidal tract dysfunction
Coordination	To a large extent assessed by gait. Ask child to slide heel of one leg along shin of other and vice versa

EXAM A

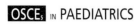

Michael, aged 7 years, is brought to hospital with a 3-day history of increasing weakness occurring about a week after a bout of an upper respiratory tract infection. He is admitted to hospital and over the next few days the weakness worsens.

On examination he has bilateral facial nerve palsies and marked weakness of both legs with loss of deep tendon reflexes. There is also mild symmetrical weakness of his arms with loss of tendon reflexes. There is no sensory deficit and no papilloedema. Abdominal examination reveals the presence of a palpable midline mass arising from the pelvis. Systems examination is otherwise normal.

1.1 In the presence of a normal cerebrospinal fluid white cell count (WCC) the most likely diagnosis is:
a. polymyositis
b. poliomyelitis
c. a spinal cord tumour
d. Guillain–Barré syndrome.

1.2 The most sensitive measure of respiratory muscle involvement is a change in:
a. arterial P_{O_2}
b. arterial CO_2
c. respiratory rate
d. peak flow measurements
e. vital capacity.

1.3 What is the midline mass, explain its significance and how should it be managed?

2.1   Give three abnormalities seen on this chest X-ray.

2.2   Through which anatomical defect does this abnormality usually occur?

2.3   What two other anatomical abnormalities are almost certainly present?

2.4   What is the diagnosis?

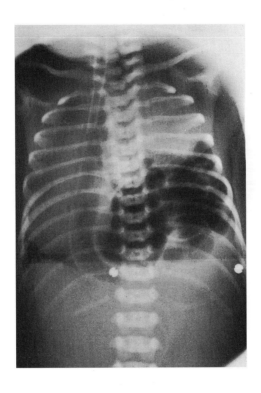

3.1   What clinical condition is shown in this slide?

3.2   What are the first signs of visual disturbance?

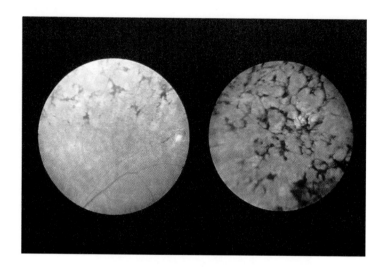

4.1 What does this picture show?

4.2 What is the diagnosis?

4.3 What two other abnormalities of the genitourinary system are commonly associated?

4.4 What surgical procedure is contraindicated?

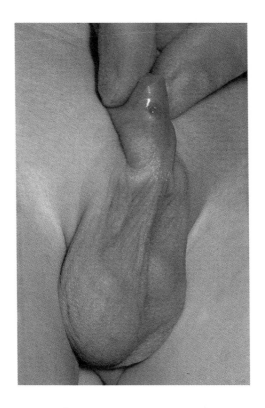

A 2-year-old boy is brought to casualty acutely unwell. A week earlier he had vomiting and diarrhoea which was beginning to settle. His parents say he has not passed much urine all day. On examination he is lethargic, pale and mildly dehydrated.

Investigations: Na (sodium) 129, K (potassium) 6, U (urea) 15, haemoglobin (Hb) 8, WCC 8, platelets (Plat) 50

5.1 What is the likely diagnosis?

5.2 What further investigations or examination would you carry out at this stage? Choose three from:
   a. Blood pressure
   b. Urinalysis
   c. Serum creatinine
   d. Renal biopsy
   e. Intravenous pyelogram
   f. Cystoscopy
   g. Blood culture.

5.3 What is the mortality rate?
   a. 10–20%
   b. 50%
   c. 60–70%
   d. 80–90%.

6.1 Describe the features on these abdominal X-rays and suggest a diagnosis and ages at which these are likely to occur.

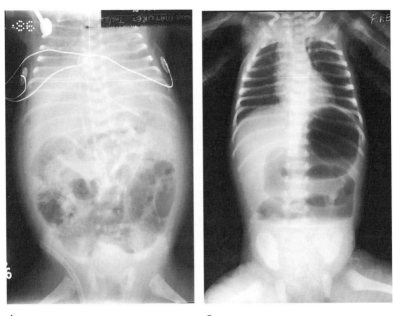

A   C

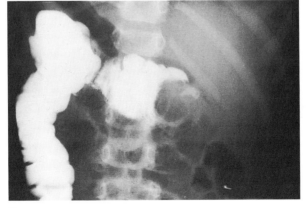

B

The photomicrographs below of a urine specimen are from a 3-year-old boy who presented with discoloured urine, poor urine output, puffy eyes and slightly raised blood pressure.

   Investigations: urine haematuria +++; protein – trace only.

7.1   What are the features on these photomicrographs?

7.2   What is the most likely diagnosis?

7.3   From the list choose the most useful investigations to perform at this stage:
     a. 24-h urine protein
     b. serum urea + electrolytes (U&E)
     c. urine microscopy, culture and sensitivity (M,C&S)
     d. throat swab
     e. renal biopsy
     f. anti-streptolysin titre (ASOT)
     g. intravenous pyelogram
     h. ultrasound scan of kidneys?

7.4   What is the prognosis? Choose one of the following:
     a. 90% improve spontaneously
     b. 40% mortality
     c. 40% develop chronic renal failure
     d. 20% mortality.

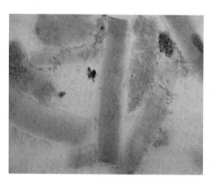 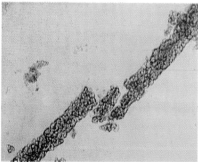

A midwife asks a doctor to see a newborn baby who she suspects to have Down syndrome.

8.1 If the midwife's observations are correct what areas of examination are of immediate concern?

8.2 Assuming the clinical diagnosis is confirmed, who should impart the news to the parents?

8.3 Who should be present?

8.4 How should information about Down syndrome be imparted? Write short notes.

8.5 What tests should be arranged?

A couple expecting their second child request information from their GP regarding prevention of cot death. Their previous baby died of this and they ask what might be done to prevent a recurrence.

9.1   What are the risk factors that you, as their GP, would inform these parents about?

Sachin, a 9-year-old boy, is brought to hospital with sudden onset of vomiting. He is from India and like his family speaks little English, having been resident in the UK for only 18 months. For the last 6 months the whole family has been treated for pulmonary tuberculosis with rifampicin and isoniazid. There had been concerns of poor compliance from the whole family and some months earlier a 21-year-old sister had died from a massive pulmonary haemorrhage secondary to active tuberculosis. Since then and unknown to the hospital the boy had been forced to take the medication despite complaints that on taking the drugs he became acutely unwell with shivers, fever and occasionally vomiting.

On examination he is unwell and has ascites with peripheral oedema. The heart is not enlarged and there are no murmurs. Respiratory examination is normal and there is no hepatosplenomegaly.

Investigations: Na 128, K 6.9, U 28, Creatinine 469.

10.1 What do the clinical findings and plasma electrolytes suggest?

10.2 Why might he have developed this complication?

11.1 What does this X-ray show?

11.2 What is the diagnosis?

11.3 At what age is this likely to present? Choose one of the following:
a. early infancy
b. late infancy
c. within the first day of life
d. early neonatal period
e. anytime in the first 2–3 years.

11.4 What is the most likely presentation?

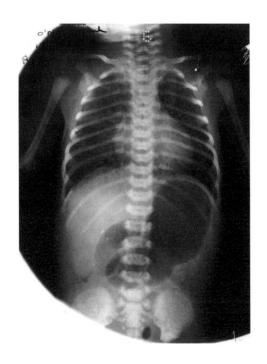

A 7-year-old asthmatic is brought into casualty acutely breathless. On examination he has marked intercostal recession with bilateral rhonchi and reduced air entry. His peak flow rate (PFR) is 35% of his normal. His normal medication includes budesonide and terbutaline, both via turbohalers, and slow-release theophylline tablets at night.

12.1 What are the first two steps in management? Choose one from the following:
   a. measure blood pressure and perform an arterial gas
   b. measure blood pressure and give nebulized salbutamol
   c. perform an arterial gas and then apply oxygen via a facemask
   d. apply oxygen and give nebulized salbutamol
   e. give nebulized salbutamol and ipratropium bromide
   f. after an arterial gas measurement give nebulized salbutamol.

5 min after one of the above steps an intravenous line is inserted and hydrocortisone given. Half an hour later he is still in marked respiratory distress although the PFR is now 50% of his normal. Nebulized salbutamol is given.

12.2 What is the next step in management? Choose one from the following:
   a. take serum for theophylline level; depending on this decide on dose of intravenous aminophylline therapy
   b. give intravenous aminophylline omitting the loading dose
   c. give intravenous salbutamol
   d. give intravenous salbutamol and intravenous aminophylline, omitting the loading dose
   e. intubate and ventilate.

12.3 Which of the following are commonly useful investigations in the acute management of asthma in children. You may choose more than one from:
   a. arterial blood gas
   b. chest X-ray
   c. pulsus paradoxus assessment
   d. none of these.

A 7-year-old boy with diabetes mellitus is admitted with a history of lethargy, polydipsia, polyuria and a fever for 3 days. On examination he has a dry tongue, sunken eyes, tachycardia, hypotension, decreased skin turgor, sighing respiration and drowsiness. He weighs 20 kg. His blood results are as follows: glucose 35, sodium 139, urea 7.5, potassium 4.0, pH 7.20, HCO_3 15.0, P_{CO_2} 5.8, base excess 9.5, WCC 24 (80% neutrophils).

13.1 Give an estimate of the degree of dehydration? Choose one of the following:
 a. less than 5%
 b. 5–10%
 c. 10–15%
 d. 20–25%

13.2 What is the first step of treatment? Choose one of the following:
 a. sodium bicarbonate to correct acidosis
 b. insulin to correct hyperglycaemia
 c. intravenous broad-spectrum antibiotics
 d. intravenous fluids to improve circulation
 e. intubation and ventilation.

13.3 Assuming the maintenance fluid requirements (including insensible losses) of this child are 70 ml/kg/day and that there are no further significant ongoing losses, calculate the fluid volume replacement therapy of the next 24 h. For the degree of dehydration (deficit) choose one of the figures from the first question – no marks will be deducted for choosing the wrong percentage at this step. Show your calculations.

14.1 What diagnosis is indicated by the abnormal pH study?

14.2 What is the most common clinical presentation of this diagnosis?

14.3 Which of the following are recognized presentations of this diagnosis?
   a. screaming attacks
   b. chronic diarrhoea
   c. recurrent pneumonia
   d. apnoeic attacks
   e. failure to thrive
   f. stridor.

14.4 Suggest two therapeutic changes that may be useful.

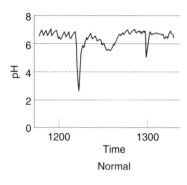

Normal

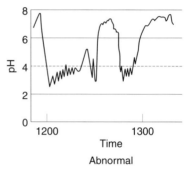

Abnormal

Sara, aged 13 months, is due her next set of immunizations. She had the first series of immunizations without complication. She is well but was admitted to hospital 3 weeks earlier following a febrile convulsion secondary to an upper respiratory tract infection.

15.1 Which diseases is Sara due to be immunized against? Her mother asks you whether there are any complications associated with the immunization.

15.2 Give two complications.

15.3 She asks if there are any severe complications. Name one.

She tells you that she is unconvinced that Sara needs immunization against these diseases.

15.4 Write short notes on what you would say to try and convince her that Sara needs immunizing.

Despite your efforts Sara's mother refuses consent for immunization.

15.5 What options are open to you in order to ensure that Sara receives her immunization?

The blood glucose profile of a 10-year-old boy with diabetes mellitus is shown below. His Hb A_{IC} is 12%. At the time of this profile his treatment was Actrapid (short acting insulin) and Monotard (long acting insulin) at the following doses and times:

	7 a.m	5 p.m
Actrapid (units)	6	3
Monotard (units)	8	5

16.1 Assuming good compliance and appropriate lifestyle and dietary management, what changes would you institute in the insulin dosage? Choose one of the following options:
- a. increase evening Monotard by 3 units (u)
- b. increase evening Monotard by 2 u and morning Actrapid by 2 u
- c. decrease evening Monotard by 2 u
- d. increase morning Actrapid by 2 u
- e. increase morning Actrapid by 2 u and Monotard by 2 u
- f. increase morning Actrapid by 2 u and decrease evening Monotard by 4 u.

16.2 Over what period is this boy's glycaemic control likely to have been unsatisfactory? Choose one of the following options:
- a. less than 1 week
- b. 1–2 weeks
- c. 3–4 weeks
- d. at least 2–3 months.

16.3 Give three long-term complications of diabetes mellitus.

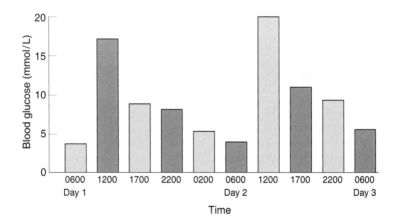

A 14-year-old girl known to have cystic fibrosis (CF) presents with a 4-day history of increasing abdominal pain and vomiting which on the last two occasions has contained bile.

On examination she has a distended abdomen with palpable loops of bowel. There is also some tenderness in the left iliac fossa but no guarding. Plain abdominal films show dilated loops of bowel with fluid levels.

17.1 Give two possible diagnoses.

17.2 Give one investigation which might help to make a diagnosis.

The audiogram below is from a 6-year-old boy with a history of recurrent upper respiratory tract infections treated with recurrent courses of antibiotics. His speech is limited but he has no other medical problems. Both his parents smoke.

18.1 At what age is pure tone audiometry possible?

18.2 What does the audiogram show?

18.3 What is the most likely diagnosis for the speech defect?

18.4 Give three steps which should be taken to help with his hearing and speech defect?

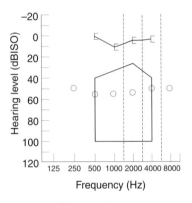

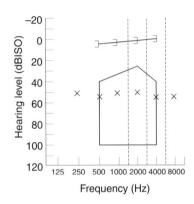

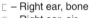

⌐ – Right ear, bone
○ – Right ear, air

⌐ – Left ear, bone
× – Left ear, air

A 13-day-old baby is admitted for excessive blood loss following circumcision. There is no family history of note.

19.1 Fill in the boxes provided with either 'increased' or 'normal' to fit with the diagnosis in the left-hand column:

	Bleeding time	PTTK	PT
Haemophilia A or B			
von Willebrand's disease			
Vitamin K deficiency			

PT, prothrombin time; PTTK, partial thromboplastin time.

This picture shows the sex chromosomes of a 13-year-old boy under investigation with normal male sex chromosomes for comparison.

20.1 What is the abnormality?

20.2 What is the diagnosis?

20.3 What clinical features may be present in the child affected with the defect? Choose any number of the following:
a. mental retardation
b. hypogonadism
c. prominent ears and mandible
d. postpubertal macro-orchidism
e. infertility
f. gynaecomastia in adolescence.

20.4 What is the usual mode of inheritance?

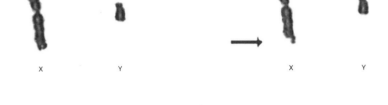

X   Y   X   Y

1.1 d

1.2 e

1.3 Michael has urinary retention which suggests autonomic nerve involvement. He needs to be catheterized.

Discussion

The history points to a symmetrical motor neuropathy without sensory nerve involvement, for which there are only a handful of acquired causes. In the UK polio is extremely rare. You would not expect a spinal cord tumour to cause facial nerve involvement. Polymyositis is a muscle disorder and tendon reflexes should be normal. From the list the diagnosis that best fits with the history is Guillain–Barré syndrome. Serial vital capacity measurements are the most sensitive means of assessing respiratory muscle involvement. However, a combination of vital capacity and peak flow measurements are usually used to monitor respiratory function.

2.1 This X-ray show a ventilated child with loops of bowel in the left hemithorax. There is also mediastinal shift to the right and absence of a gastric bubble.

2.2 The diaphragm forms through the fusion of the pleuro-peritoneal membranes. Most large hernias pass through an anterior defect where the *foramen of Bochdalek* would normally form.

2.3 A hypoplastic left lung and malrotation of the bowel.

2.4 Left congenital diaphragmatic hernia.

Discussion

Congenital diaphragmatic hernia is one of the commonest thoracoabdominal emergencies and is associated with a high mortality. Its incidence is approximately 1 in 3000 and 90% are left sided. Other associated conditions include congenital heart disease and lobar sequestration. Most diagnoses are now made on antenatal ultrasound scan.

Whereas previously surgical repair was carried out within hours of diagnosis, it is now recommended that for the best results there is a period, often of days, where preoperative intensive medical stabilization is carried out. This includes early and constant nasogastric suctioning to prevent intrathoracic gastrointestinal distension. Acidosis is treated vigorously and oxygenation improved. Ventilation can include conventional or high-frequency oscillation. Inhaled nitric oxide and increasingly extracorporeal membranous oxygenation are used in severe cases where pulmonary hypertension is a particular problem.

3.1 Retinitis pigmentosa.

3.2 Loss of night vision.

Discussion
The bone corpuscle pattern is due to pigment deposition in the retina and is characteristic of retinitis pigmentosa. This is a progressive disorder eventually leading to blindness. The earliest sign of this is loss of night vision. It can be an isolated disease with a variable inheritance pattern or it may be part of a syndrome such as the Laurence–Moon–Biedl syndrome (polydactyly, obesity and mental retardation).

4.1 Urethral meatal opening on the ventral surface of the penis at the base of the glans.

4.2 Hypospadias.

4.3 Urinary tract abnormalities and undescended testicles.

4.4 Circumcision.

Discussion
Hypospadias is commonly associated with chordee (ventral curvature of the penis) and a hooded prepuce (deficiency of the ventral foreskin). Circumcision is absolutely contraindicated as the prepuce is used for surgical repair of the hypospadias which is normally carried out at 1 year of age. Other associated conditions include: urinary tract abnormalities (e.g. horseshoe kidney, reflux), congenital adrenal hyperplasia, hermaphroditism and undescended testicles.

5.1 Haemolytic uraemic syndrome

5.2 a, b and c

5.3 a

Discussion
Haemolytic uraemic syndrome, although rare, is serious in that there is a 10–20% mortality. Oliguria, oedema and a bleeding tendency (petechiae) with pallor and sometimes jaundice are the presenting features. Acute renal failure and fluid overload can lead to severe hypertension and secondary complications, including heart failure and convulsions. It tends to occur in the 6–36-month age group, often following an episode of gastroenteritis. The clinical picture and finding red cell fragments (haemolysis) in the blood is

often enough to confirm the diagnosis. Urinalysis, monitoring blood pressure and serum creatinine are useful investigations at this stage.

STATION 6 ANSWERS **EXAM A**

6.1 A. Dilated loops of bowel, pneumatosis coli – air in bowel wall, translucent streaks in right lower quadrant and large central air shadow. A nasogastric tube and ECG leads are present.
Diagnosis – necrotizing enterocolitis with perforation. This occurs in the neonatal period.

B. Barium flow obstructed by a mass with a concave appearance is shown in this contrast barium enema. Some barium has passed beyond the obstruction giving a coiled-spring appearance to the bowel.
Diagnosis – intussusception. This occurs in infancy.

C. Dilated gastric shadow and loops of small bowel. Fluid levels are present. No gas is present in the large bowel.
Diagnosis – small bowel obstruction. This usually presents in the neonatal period.

STATION 7 ANSWERS **EXAM A**

7.1 Hyaline and red cell casts.

7.2 Acute glomerulonephritis.

7.3 a, b, c, d and f

7.4 a

Discussion
The presence of hyaline and red cell casts with a history of periorbital oedema, oliguria and haematuria is characteristic of acute glomerulonephritis. In childhood this is most commonly associated with a preceding streptococcal infection, usually of the throat. Complications include acute renal failure leading to hyperkalaemia, hypertension and fluid overload. Serum U&E, creatinine, blood pressure and weight need to be regularly monitored. Urine must be sent for C&S to exclude urinary tract infection. Throat swab, complement and ASOT would be useful to try and confirm the aetiology of the glomerulonephritis. A 24-h urinary protein will help exclude the nephrotic syndrome. The other investigations listed would not be as useful during this stage of the management. Prognosis is good, with approximately 90% improving spontaneously.

STATION 8 ANSWERS **EXAM A**

8.1 Particular attention should be paid to examination of the eyes (increased risk of cataract and congenital glaucoma), the

OSCEs IN PAEDIATRICS

gastrointestinal tract and the heart (40% have some form of congenital heart disease).

8.2 Ideally, a doctor who is familiar to the parents and has been taught or had direct experience of imparting such news.

8.3 The mother, the father (a close relative if father not available), a key nurse/health visitor and the baby.

8.4 Information should be imparted over two or three meetings. Attention to language is vital. Refer to the baby by name. It is important to create a positive but not over optimistic appraisal of the ability of people with Down syndrome. Written information including the address of the Down Syndrome Association is also useful.

8.5 Karyotype and echocardiography.

Discussion
It is important to know that the trisomy occurred because of non-dysjunction at meiosis (90% of cases) rather than because one of the parents is a carrier of a balanced translocation involving chromosome 21 (10% of cases), where the recurrence risk is higher. Echocardiography is essential despite the absence of clinical signs of a cardiac anomaly.

STATION 9	ANSWERS	EXAM A

9.1 The modifiable risk factors are:

- Sleeping position – recent evidence suggests that a change in the sleeping position from prone to supine can reduce the mortality from 30% to 70%. This is the most important risk factor recognized up until now.
- Smoking – not only maternal but also paternal smoking is associated with cot death.
- Thermal insulation – excessive swaddling and sleeping in rooms with excessive heating have also been recognized as significant risk factors.
- Breast feeding reduces the incidence of cot death compared to bottle feeding, even when allowance is made for social class.

Less easily or non-modifiable risk factors include:

- Colder geographic regions.
- Fetal growth retardation.
- Low socioeconomic status.
- Young maternal age.
- Lower levels of education.
- Recent illness.
- Less use of preventive health services, e.g. antenatal care.

Apnoea alarms are often requested from GPs by parents in this situation. There is, however, no evidence that these are of benefit.

10.1 Acute renal failure.

10.2 Allergy to rifampicin.

Discussion

This case highlights some of the problems associated with treating serious diseases with potentially dangerous drugs without effective monitoring. Most patients/parents would have been able to communicate the side effects and would have alerted the physician. The combination of poor communication (language), a death in the family and, perhaps, previous accusations of poor compliance have all contributed to this child being forced to take a drug to which he is obviously allergic. As a consequence he has developed renal failure. The most likely drug to have caused this problem is rifampicin.

11.1 'Double-bubble', air in the proximal duodenum and the stomach.

11.2 Duodenal stenosis or atresia.

11.3 c

11.4 Bile-stained vomiting.

Discussion

This is the X-ray appearance of a duodenal stenosis or atresia. A 'double-bubble' indicates air accumulation in the proximal duodenum and the stomach. Note that there are no distal gas shadows. This diagnosis should be suspected in any pregnancy complicated by polyhydramnios. Newborns usually present with bile-stained vomiting within the first 24 h of birth with little or no abdominal distension and normal passage of meconium. Duodenal atresia/stenosis are associated with Down syndrome. In non-syndromic cases other congenital abnormalities, e.g. heart and renal anomalies, may be present. The definitive treatment is surgical repair.

12.1 d

12.2 b or c

12.3 d

Discussion

Any asthmatic with a PFR almost a third of normal is in a life-threatening state and needs immediate treatment. In the first instance nebulized salbutamol and oxygen are essential; if the response is inadequate the salbutamol dose can be repeated with or without ipratropium bromide

OSCEs IN PAEDIATRICS

(Atrovent), also via a nebulizer. During the acute stage of a severe asthma exacerbation in children arterial blood gases (ABG), chest X-ray (CXR) and pulsus paradoxus assessment are unnecessary and rarely helpful. ABG may be useful if the child is not responding or deteriorating despite treatment. CXRs may be helpful in rare circumstances when collapse of a lobe of lung or a pneumothorax is clinically suspected. Corticosteroid therapy is almost always indicated when asthma is this severe. If despite this there is still inadequate recovery or deterioration, then intravenous bronchodilator therapy is required. As this child was already on theophylline, omitting the loading dose and starting with a maintenance dose is recommended. Intravenous salbutamol is being increasingly used and is an acceptable alternative to aminophylline, and especially in a case such as this, when the child is already on theophylline. ECG monitoring would be essential when either of these drugs are given. Rarely, the combined use of intravenous salbutamol and aminophylline is required and can prevent the need for ventilation. Starting both of these together is not recommended. Serum electrolytes need to be checked regularly, as salbutamol causes hypokalaemia.

STATION 13	ANSWERS	EXAM A

13.1 c

13.2 d

13.3 120 ml/h – see text

Discussion

Diabetic ketoacidosis usually presents with the above features, nausea, vomiting and smell of ketones in the breath. It may be triggered by an upper respiratory tract infection. Unless a very recent weight is available the degree of dehydration is assessed by the features mentioned in the history. The presence of the features in this case indicate a dehydration level of approximately *10–15 %*. This child is clearly in shock and the immediate treatment is to *improve the circulation* by giving 20 ml/kg of colloid/crystalloid.

The subsequent fluid replacement is based on replacing the deficit and providing the maintenance at the same time. Fluid deficit approximates to $15/100 \times 20\,000$ ml (assuming 15% dehydration and a weight of 20 kg) – this equals 3000 ml. Maintenance is 70×20 (using 70 ml/kg/day as the maintenance and 20 kg as weight) – this equals 1400 ml. The deficit is normally replaced over 48 h; therefore 1500 ml needs to be replaced over the first 24 h. The total volume to be given over the first 24 h is 1500 plus 1400 ml – this equals 2900 ml. This equates to $2900/24 = 120$ *ml per hour*. 0.45% saline, 4% dextrose is a suitable replacement fluid for the first 24 h. Repeat serum electrolytes and acid-base balance will guide subsequent therapy. Fluid replacement is carried out slowly to reduce rapid osmotic shifts and hence the risk of complications, e.g. cerebral oedema. Sodium bicarbonate is only rarely required; replacing the fluid deficit usually normalizes the pH. Insulin treatment is however essential and is usually commenced with the maintenance fluid therapy. Intravenous potassium is usually given when it is confirmed that the serum level is not raised and the urinary output has returned. Antibiotics should only be given when bacterial infection is thought likely or proven from culture results.

| STATION 14 | ANSWERS | EXAM A |

14.1 Gastro-oesophageal reflux.

14.2 Vomiting.

14.3 a, c, d and e

14.4 Thickening milk feeds, Gaviscon, cisapride or H_2 blocker.

Discussion

Gastro-oesophageal reflux most commonly presents with regurgitation of feeds in the first few days of life which may progress on to recurrent vomiting. This may lead to aspiration pneumonia as well as vagus nerve-mediated bradycardia and apnoea. Secondary oesophagitis may cause irritability, screaming attacks and blood loss, leading to iron deficiency anaemia. Severe reflux can lead to failure to thrive. A 24-h ambulatory oesophageal pH study, showing greater than 4% of a 24-h period with the pH less than 4, is currently the most sensitive investigation. Barium studies, radioisotope milk scans and endoscopy are also useful for diagnosis.

Management involves: increasing the time spent in an upright position (babychair, sleeping in 30° head-up position), thickening feeds (e.g. Carobel, addition of Gaviscon, H_2 blocker – if suggested by the pH study), and, in severe cases, cisapride to increase the lower oesophageal sphincter pressure and enhance gastric emptying. Surgical treatment (Nissen's fundoplication) is reserved for patients unresponsive to medical treatment.

| STATION 15 | ANSWERS | EXAM A |

15.1 Measles, Mumps and Rubella (MMR).

15.2 Fever, febrile convulsions.

15.3 Yes, post immunization meningoencephalomyelitis. These questions should be approached with candour, although the answer should be phrased in terms of the complications associated with the three diseases. Severe complications include: measles – acute encephalitis and in the long term subacute sclerosing panencephalitis (SSPE); mumps – deafness and acute encephalitis; rubella – acute encephalitis. All viral encephalitides are associated with CNS damage. Finally you should say that the complications associated with the immunization are similar to those found in the individual diseases but less severe and 10–100 times less common and that immunization protects against SSPE.

OSCEs IN PAEDIATRICS

15.4 This problem is not uncommon. To convince parents that their child needs immunization against diseases that are perceived as trivial can be difficult. It is best to admit these three diseases are usually not life threatening. However, you should quickly move on to saying that there is a small but significant number of children who develop severe complications *every year*. Knowing a few short-term problems and long-term complications associated with each disease will convince most of the necessity for the immunization.

15.5 Offer an appointment with the district immunization officer or paediatrician. At the end of the day the parents are free to say no.

STATION 16 ANSWERS · EXAM A

16.1 d

16.2 d

16.3 Hypertension, ischaemic heart disease and nephropathy.

Discussion
In an otherwise well diabetic the blood glucose will be determined by energy expenditure, caloric intake and the dose of insulin. In this case the first two are appropriate for age. Normoglycaemia can only be achieved in these circumstances by altering the dosage of insulin. This boy's blood glucose profile is consistently high at midday. The insulin having the predominant effect at this time is the morning Actrapid. The most appropriate action to take is, therefore, to increase the dose of this by 2 u in the morning.

Glycosylated haemoglobin, Hb A$_{1C}$, reflects the approximate average of the blood glucose concentrations over the preceding 2–3 months. Values of 6–9% represent very good control and 9–12% fair control.

Preventable long-term complications of diabetes include diabetic nephropathy, retinopathy, neuropathy, ischaemic heart disease and hypertension.

STATION 17 ANSWERS · EXAM A

17.1 Distal intestinal obstruction syndome (DIOS) and intussusception.

17.2 Abdominal ultrasound or gastrograffin enema.

Discussion
The most likely diagnosis is distal intestinal obstruction syndrome, which results from inspissated faeces/mucus in the terminal ileum and colon and is analogous to meconium ileus in newborns with CF. Intussusception, fibrosing colonopathy – an intestinal stricture thought to be associated with pancreatic enzyme replacement therapy – and volvulus can all cause bowel obstruction and must be considered in the differential diagnosis. All of these are more common in children with CF. The most useful investigations would include an

abdominal ultrasound and gastrograffin enema. A barium enema is contraindicated in a surgical abdomen where intestinal perforation may be present, as it may allow leak of barium into the peritoneum and lead to a chemical peritonitis.

STATION 18 ANSWERS   EXAM A

18.1 5 years.

18.2 Bilateral conductive hearing loss.

18.3 Serous bilateral otitis media.

18.4 This is usually managed with grommet insertion. Other important steps which will help his speech delay include sitting at the front of the class, reducing cigarette smoke exposure and speech therapy.

Discussion
Children under 4 are unlikely to understand and/or cooperate sufficiently to perform pure tone audiometry. It is possible to perform tests in nearly all children over 5 years. This audiogram shows normal bone conduction but moderate bilateral hearing loss, indicating conductive hearing loss. A speech defect with conductive hearing loss suggests chronic middle ear problems. All the management options mentioned above can be usefully employed to improve this child's speech defect and improve his ability to learn at school.

STATION 19 ANSWERS   EXAM A

19.1

	Bleeding time	PTTK	PT
Haemophilia A or B	normal	increased	normal
von Willebrand's disease	increased	increased	normal
Vitamin K deficiency	normal	increased	increased

Discussion
Haemophilia A and B are due to deficiencies in Factor VIII and Factor IX respectively. Both result in a prolonged PTTK and no other abnormalities on coagulation studies. von Willebrand's disease is due to deficiency of a serum factor termed von Willebrand's factor which promotes platelet adhesiveness and prevents destruction of Factor VIII. Hence affected individuals exhibit platelet aggregation abnormalities (prolonged bleeding time) and a prolonged PTTK. Vitamin K deficiency results in a reduced production of hepatic Vitamin K-dependent coagulation factors (II, VII, IX and X) and results in prolonged PTTK and PT.

OSCEs IN PAEDIATRICS

20.1 Defect in the long arm of the X chromosome.

20.2 Fragile X syndrome.

20.3 a, c and d

20.4 X-linked recessive.

Discussion

Fragile X syndrome is the commonest genetic cause of severe learning difficulty after Down syndrome. Prevalence is in the region of 0.5–1 in 1000 males. There is usually a defect or gap in the distal part of the long arm of the X chromosome. Currently, the diagnosis has been greatly improved by DNA analysis of the affected gene, and has been used for carrier detection and antenatal diagnosis.

The majority of children have moderate learning difficulties – IQ is approximately 20–80. Other features include macrocephaly and postpubertal testicular enlargement. The facial features of long face, large forehead, prominent ears and mandible are usually more evident in affected adults. Infertility and gynaecomastia are not features of this condition – compare with Klinefelter syndrome.

The usual mode of inheritance is X-linked recessive. A large proportion of the female carriers have, however, mild learning difficulties and nearly 20% of males who have inherited the mutation are phenotypically normal. The latter may pass the defect to grandsons via their daughters.

EXAM B

A previously well 14-year-old girl is brought into casualty unconscious. Her teacher reports that she was acting strangely in class half an hour prior to collapsing. She has an 8-year-old brother with diabetes mellitus and her father is on treatment for epilepsy.

On examination she is apyrexial and there are no rashes. Her pulse rate is 70/min, BP 110/80 and respiratory rate 18/min. She does respond to pain and fundoscopy is normal.

1.1 From the following list select the five most useful investigations and one investigation that is contraindicated.
  a. chest X-ray
  b. blood sugar
  c. lumbar puncture
  d. gastric washout
  e. urine for toxicology
  f. arterial blood gases
  g. erythrocyre sedimentation rate (ESR)
  h. urine culture
  i. U&E.

A 10-month-old infant had been fitting for about 10 min with tonic-clonic movements before being seen in casualty. Over the last 24 h he had been non-specifically unwell with mild pyrexia, vomiting and lethargy. There is no past history of note.

2.1 Which two of the following combinations of anticonvulsants could be used at this stage?
  a. diazepam followed by paraldehyde
  b. diazepam followed by chlormethiazole
  c. phenytoin followed by phenobarbitone
  d. diazepam followed by phenytoin
  e. phenobarbitone followed by chlormethiazole
  f. clonazepam followed by phenytoin.

The blood sugar is 5 and the temperature is 38.5°C. Within 5 min of one of the above steps the fit stops. On examination he is drowsy but with no obvious focus of infection. Rectal paracetamol is given.

2.2 What is the most appropriate action to take at this stage? Choose one from the list below:
  a. perform a full blood count, blood culture and C-reactive protein (CRP); if any of these suggest a significant bacterial infection then proceed to a full sepsis screen (i.e. lumbar puncture (LP), CXR, urine microscopy, C&S and throat swab, etc.) with the appropriate treatment
  b. a full sepsis screen followed by appropriate treatment
  c. perform a limited sepsis screen without an LP
  d. perform a limited sepsis screen as in c, but immediately follow with broad-spectrum intravenous antibiotics even if the results are negative.

2.3 Assuming that no cause other than an upper respiratory tract infection (URTI) was found, what is the risk of further febrile convulsions and what advice would you give to parents regarding management of subsequent febrile episodes?

This EEG record is from a 5-month-old infant who episodically raises his arms and then flexes his neck, trunk and hips. The episodes last a few seconds and end with a brief cry and return to a normal posture. The episodes occur in quick succession with several hours passing between each cluster of attacks.

3.1   What does the EEG show?

3.2   What syndrome is suggested by the history and EEG?

3.3   Give one condition associated with this syndrome.

3.4   What is the long-term prognosis? Choose one of the following:
    a. death usually within 2 years
    b. long-term developmental delay and in some cases regression
    c. the majority show gradual developmental progress
    d. death usually within 5 years
    e. developmental delay, but with an improvement in epilepsy.

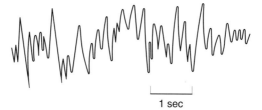

1 sec

The photograph shows the hands of a child who has had an unremitting fever for 10 days. He is noted to have bilateral conjunctivitis, non-suppurative cervical lymphadenopathy, pharyngeal inflammation and a generalized polymorphous erythematous rash. His full blood count shows: Hb 12, WCC 20, Plat 900.

4.1 What is the most likely diagnosis?

4.2 What is the most serious complication?

4.3 What is the treatment of choice?

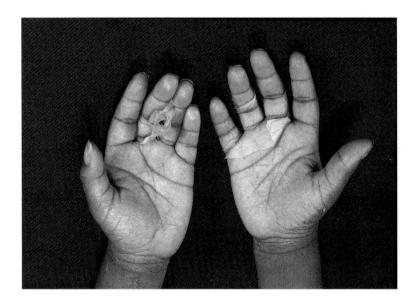

A 3-year-old child presents with a 1-week history of intermittent fever and general malaise after returning 2 weeks ago from a 4-week holiday in Nigeria. He is not systemically unwell and no foci of infection can be found. Full blood count shows a Hb of 9 and a WCC of 8.

5.1 Name three investigations that you would carry out.

5.2 What diagnosis must be excluded?

5.3 What steps can be taken to prevent this?

This is the growth chart of a boy who has normal neurological development.

6.1   Give two possible diagnoses.

6.2   What is the most likely diagnosis?

6.3   Name three long-term complications of the most likely diagnosis.

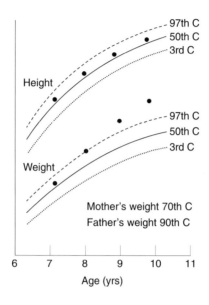

7.1 What are the four development milestones shown in these pictures?

7.2 At what ages are these normally developed?

7.3 How old do you think this child is?

7.4 What is the expected speech development at this age?

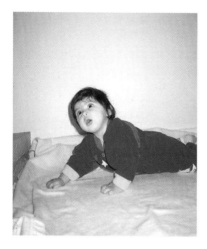 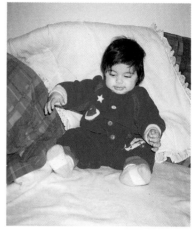

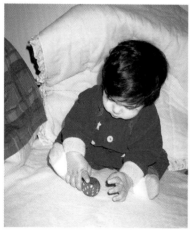 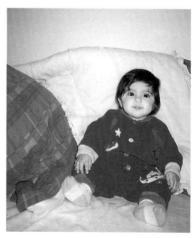

These are the X-rays of a 2-day-old term baby admitted to neonatal intensive care with a history of abdominal distension with bilious vomiting and never having passed meconium.

8.1 What features are present on these X-rays?

8.2 What is the likely diagnosis?

8.3 Give two tests that might be useful in confirming the underlying diagnosis.

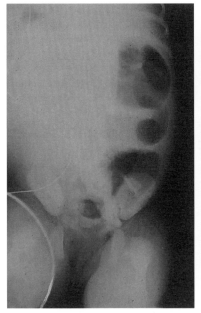
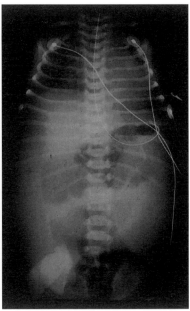

A 15-year-old girl presents with a history of lethargy, weight loss and abdominal pain. At school she has not been able to concentrate or take part in physical exercise and has been having episodes of dizziness.

On examination she has two hypopigmented patches on her left forearm, but in general she appears hyperpigmented especially on her appendix scar. Her pulse is 70/min and BP 110 /80 supine and 90/70 erect.

Investigations: Na 128, K 6.5, Urea 7, Ca 2.4 and fasting glucose 2.

9.1   Suggest two causes for the dizzy episodes.

9.2   What is the likely diagnosis?

Sharon, aged 8 years, is referred by her GP to the local hospital, having developed an anorectal fistula. Over the last 6 months she has been to see her GP three times, complaining of a sore mouth. Her parents say she has not been herself, being lethargic with a poor appetite. They have attributed this to a recent move to a new area and school. Over the past week she has had abdominal pain associated with diarrhoea occasionally tinged with blood.

On examination she is pale with a temperature of 38°C. There is diffuse abdominal tenderness with no guarding. Rectal examination reveals a fistulous opening; internal examination is not performed.

She has lesions in her mouth, as shown on the photograph below.

10.1 What are these lesions?

10.2 What is the most likely diagnosis?

10.3 What further tests are needed to help manage Sharon's illness? Choose three out of the following:
a. colonoscopy and biopsy
b. barium studies
c. stool culture
d. technetium scanning
e. CT scan of abdomen.

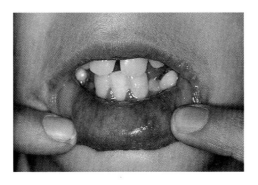

The DMSA scan below is of an 8-month-old infant with a history of recurrent urinary tract infections (UTI).

11.1 What are the features of this scan?

11.2 What does this signify?

11.3 What other renal investigations would be helpful? Choose one of the following combinations:
   a. ultrasound (US) and micturating cystourethrogram (MCUG)
   b. creatinine clearance and MCUG
   c. glomerular filtration rate (GFR) and US
   d. creatinine clearance and DTPA scan
   e. US and intravenous urography (IVU)
   f. DTPA scan and IVU.

11.4 What cardiovascular complication needs to be monitored?

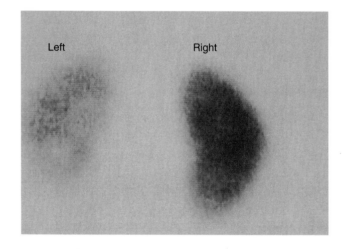

12.1 An 8-year-old girl is referred for chronic headaches. What relevant history would you take to try and arrive at a diagnosis? Write the history in note form.

13.1 Describe the most prominent features on these X-rays and suggest a diagnosis for each.

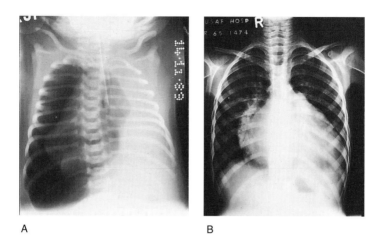

A

B

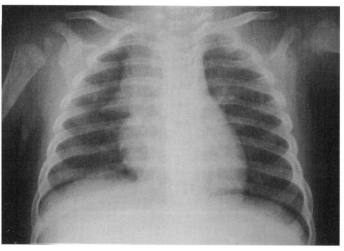

C

An 11-year-old girl with cystic fibrosis is found on routine assessment to be pale and have an enlarged liver and spleen.
Investigations: Hb 9, WCC 2, Plat 56, liver enzymes moderately raised.

14.1 What complication of CF has this girl developed?

14.2 What is the likely cause for the thrombocytopenia?

14.3 What proportion of patients affected with CF develop this complication? Choose one of the following:
a. >90%
b. 50–90%
c. all will eventually
d. <10%.

This boy presented with acute abdominal pain radiating to the testes.

15.1 Give two possible diagnoses.

15.2 What is the management?

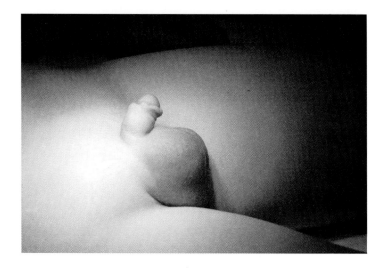

     OSCEs ɪɴ PAEDIATRICS

John, aged 9 years, had surgery for tetralogy of Fallot 10 months ago. For the last 3 weeks he has been treated with topical and oral antibiotics for a toe nail paronychia. He presents to the local hospital with a 24-h history of becoming increasingly unwell and has been unable to move his left leg for the past hour.

On examination he has a severe episode of shivering associated with a high temperature. Several macular skin lesions are noted on the soles of his feet which do not blanch on pressure. A loud pan-systolic murmur is heard all over the precordium. Flaccid paralysis of the left leg with diminished ankle and knee tendon reflexes and an extensor plantar reflex are present. Fundoscopy is normal.

16.1 What further investigations would you perform at this stage? Choose three of the following:
   a. blood culture
   b. urine M,C&S
   c. CRP
   d. echocardiogram
   e. ECG
   f. cranial computed tomography (CT) scan.

16.2 What are the skin lesions described and name two other skin manifestations of this disease?

16.3 Where is the lesion causing the neurological abnormality?

16.4 What is the diagnosis?

17.1 What is the diagnosis?

17.2 What features might be associated with this?

17.3 What is the presurgical management?

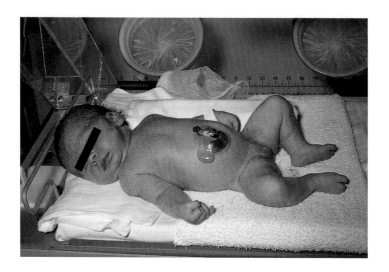

A paediatrician is asked to attend a delivery as there have been some type 2 dips on the cardiotocograph. The mother has been in the second stage of labour for 15 min and had been given intramuscular pethidine 45 min ago. The baby is brought to the resuscitaire and some mucus is sucked out from the oropharynx with little reaction. He is apnoeic, blue, with a heart rate of 120 and has normal tone.

18.1 Answer 'true' or 'false':

    a. heat loss is rapid in newborns and will aggravate apnoea

    b. the baby is most likely apnoeic because of maternal opiate administration; this may be reversed with naloxone

    c. the baby should be given facemask ventilation using oxygen at a rate of 40–60 breaths per min

    d. the baby is asphyxiated and requires immediate intubation

    e. oropharyngeal suction may cause bradycardia.

A 1-year-old Asian infant presents with jaundice and passing dark urine 24 h after starting antibiotics for acute otitis media. He had been unwell with the ear infection but he has become even more lethargic with the onset of jaundice.

Investigations: Hb 4.7, WCC 23, Plat 570, urine dipstick positive for haemoglobin and urobilinogen.

The following statements are true:

19.1 Spherocytes on a blood film confirm a diagnosis of hereditary spherocytosis (HS).

19.2 Antioxidant drugs may precipitate haemolytic crises in glucose-6-phosphate dehydrogenase deficiency (G6PD).

19.3 Red cells from patients with HS spontaneously rupture in the presence of hypertonic saline and form the basis of the osmotic fragility test.

19.4 The most likely diagnosis is an allergy to penicillin.

19.5 Parvovirus infections may trigger acute aplastic crisis in HS, β-thalassaemia major and in sickle cell disease.

Which feed/supplement is most useful in the conditions listed below.

Feed/supplement:
a. Maxijul
b. Galactomin 17
c. Carobel
d. Pregestimil
e. Wysoy
f. SMA – low birth weight

Condition

20.1 Cows' milk protein allergy.

20.2 Prolonged diarrhoea of unknown origin.

20.3 Intrauterine growth retardation.

20.4 Ventricular septal defect with cardiac failure and failure to thrive.

20.5 Galactosaemia.

20.6 Gastro-oesophageal reflux.

1.1   b, d, e, f and i

Lumbar puncture is contraindicated.

Discussion

Acute drug overdose is the most likely explanation for this girl's condition. Both insulin and anticonvulsant medication could induce these signs and symptoms. Alternatively she may have taken other drugs. A lumbar puncture is contraindicated because the intracranial pressure may be raised. This is despite normal fundoscopy. Meningitis must, however, be considered in the differential diagnosis and treatment with broad-spectrum antibiotics started empirically.

Gastric washout should be performed, not only for diagnosis but also for therapy. However, this should only be done after her airway has been protected by the insertion of a cuffed endotracheal tube.

2.1   a or d

2.2   b or d

2.3   See text.

Discussion

Intravenous or rectal diazepam is the first-line therapy for febrile convulsions. If maximum dosage of this does not terminate the convulsion, than rectal paraldehyde, intravenous phenytoin or phenobarbitone would be acceptable second-line medication. Chlormethiazole and clonazepam are normally reserved for convulsions not responding to the above.

Meningitis can be rapidly fatal and its classical signs – neck stiffness, rigidity and Kernig's sign – are often not present at this age. An LP and the remainder of the full sepsis screen followed by the appropriate antibiotic treatment is the preferred option. Drowsiness could be due to the effects of anticonvulsants, the postictal state or due to raised intracranial pressure secondary to meningitis. As there is a small risk of coning when performing an LP in a child with significantly raised intracranial pressure, a reasonable option is to carry out limited sepsis screen without an LP and start broad-spectrum intravenous antibiotics even if the screen results are negative.

The risk of further episodes of febrile convulsion is increased to about 5%. Future episodes of fever should be treated with: gentle sponging with tepid water, removing excess clothing and earlier and regular use of antipyretics. GP opinion should be sought if the temperature does not settle with the above.

3.1 Hypsarrhythmia.

3.2 Infantile spasms – West syndrome.

3.3 Tuberous sclerosis.

3.4 b

Discussion

The EEG shows hypsarrhythmia – large amplitude slow wave activity mixed with multifocal spikes and sharp waves which is characteristic of West syndrome (infantile spasms). This form of epilepsy always starts in the first year of life and is unmistakable when episodes are clearly described as above. The attacks are especially frequent on waking and occur in bursts several times a day. The majority of infants are developmentally delayed at diagnosis. West syndrome is associated with tuberous sclerosis, congenital infections, e.g. rubella, and birth asphyxia.

Treatment remains unsatisfactory. Vigabatrin, a new anticonvulsant, has been shown to be more efficacious than steroids and clonazepam. The long-term prognosis is largely dependent on the underlying condition. On the whole, however, most infants will have further development delay, loss of skills and continuing epilepsy. The prognosis is better for those with no underlying disorder.

4.1 Kawasaki disease.

4.2 Coronary artery aneurysms.

4.3 Immunoglobulins and antiplatelet therapy (aspirin).

Discussion

Prolonged fever of greater than 5 days, bilateral non-purulent conjunctivitis, stomatitis (strawberry tongue), lymphadenopathy (especially cervical) and generalized erythematous polymorphous rash with oedema of the hands and feet are characteristic of Kawasaki disease. Perungal desquamation (peeling of the extremities) and thrombocythaemia are late features. The diagnosis needs to be made before the latter features develop in order for the treatment to have an effect on the mortality. This is around 1–2% and is caused by the development of coronary artery aneurysms. The current recommended treatment is intravenous immunoglobulin (to prevent aneurysm formation) and aspirin (to prevent thrombosis).

Echocardiograms are used to monitor the presence and development of aneurysms and also to decide the duration of antiplatelet therapy.

5.1 Blood film looking for malarial parasites, blood culture and urine for M,C&S.

5.2 Malaria.

5.3 Malaria prophylactic medication (see text).

Discussion
Any child with a history of pyrexia of unknown origin after travel to malaria endemic areas must have a thick blood film looked at for malarial parasites. The clinical features of diarrhoea, vomiting, jaundice, splenomegaly and rigors are often not present. Although the infection usually develops 7–10 days after inoculation, it can present weeks to months later. Children are particularly susceptible to the severe form of the disease, cerebral malaria; a high index of suspicion is therefore required in these circumstances. Repeat blood films may be necessary. Other useful initial investigations to carry out include: CRP, ESR, urine for microscopy, culture and sensitivity and a blood culture. The current chemoprophylactic recommendation is for the antimalarial to be taken 1 week before travel, during it and, it must be stressed, for 4–6 weeks after return from the endemic area. Prevention of mosquito bites with repellants and bed nets is also important.

6.1 Simple obesity and Cushing's disease.

6.2 Simple obesity.

6.3 Ischaemic heart disease, maturity onset diabetes mellitus and hypertension.

Discussion
The two most likely causes of excessive weight gain in childhood are simple obesity and Cushing's disease. Other causes include hypothyroidism and Prader–Willi syndrome. In Cushing's disease, the height is usually compromised. The most likely diagnosis here is therefore simple obesity.

Obesity is linked to ischaemic heart disease, maturity onset diabetes and hypertension. The psychological effects of being teased with the subsequent adverse effects on self-confidence can be a significant problem. Severe obesity can also lead to the Pickwickian syndrome – hypoventilation and hypercapnia leading to somnolence and heart failure.

7.1, 7.2 Sitting up with support   6 months

Smiling	6 weeks
Palmar grasp	6–7 months
Lifting head and body off floor with weight on hands	4–5 months

7.3   6 months (5–7 months acceptable)

7.4   'Goo' and 'ga' – laughs, monosyllable sounds

Discussion

The ability to perform a development assessment is specific, as well as essential, to paediatric practice. Common milestones should be learnt. Some other examples are:

6 weeks	smiling, follows face in 90° arc, stills to mother's voice
4 months	rolls over front to back
6 months	palmar grasp, sits up with support, turns to voice
7–9 months	pulls self to stand
18 months	puts two words together, kicks ball, spoon feeds self

| **STATION 8** | ANSWERS | **EXAM B** |

8.1   Dilated loops of small bowel and fluid levels.

8.2   Meconium ileus syndrome.

8.3   Sweat test, immunoreactive trypsin or CF gene testing.

Discussion

10% of infants with cystic fibrosis (CF) present in the newborn period with meconium ileus syndrome. The presentation is similar to any other cause of small intestinal obstruction. The terminal ileum and colon are small, collapsed and filled with inspissated mucus. This baby needs a sweat test but a raised immunoreactive trypsin in the first 6 weeks of life is strongly suggestive of CF.

| **STATION 9** | ANSWERS | **EXAM B** |

9.1   Postural hypotension or hypoglycaemia.

9.2   Addison's disease.

Discussion

This girl has features of hypoadrenalism; postural hypotension, low sodium, raised potassium and fasting hypoglycaemia. The dizzy episodes may be related to the postural blood pressure changes or hypoglycaemia. The depigmentation suggests vitiligo and hyperpigmentation indicates increased pituitary production of adrenocorticotrophin. These features strongly suggest end-organ failure and a diagnosis of Addison's disease.

10.1 Aphthous ulcers.

10.2 Crohn's disease.

10.3 a, b, c

Discussion

This presentation is typical of childhood Crohn's disease. Non-specific symptoms such as lethargy and poor appetite become important in the context of poor weight gain and abdominal pain. Crohn's disease affects the whole of the gastrointestinal tract from the mouth to the anus. In the early stages a persistently raised ESR may be the only finding. However, untreated the disease invariably progresses to the clinical picture illustrated by this case. Diagnosis is based on barium studies/white cell scan findings and should be confirmed with a biopsy. Treatment depends on the state of the disease in which severe exacerbations are interspersed with periods of remission. During an exacerbation a low residue diet, systemic and topical steroids may be necessary, as well as supportive therapy such as blood transfusion.

11.1 Decreased isotope uptake by the left kidney generally as well as a localized decrease in uptake at the lower pole.

11.2 Scarring of the left kidney particularly localized at the lower pole.

11.3 a

11.4 Hypertension.

Discussion

Scarring implies significant damage to the kidney; in this age group the commonest cause is UTI. It may lead to chronic renal failure and hypertension. MCUG should be carried out to look for vesicoureteric reflux – the most common renal tract abnormality predisposing to UTI. US will provide a good non-invasive assessment of kidney size and anatomical defects predisposing to UTIs. GFR and creatinine clearance have almost no role to play in assessment of renal function at this age group. DTPA gives information on renal blood flow, renal function and drainage; it would normally be used when one of the above investigations suggests an abnormality of one of these. IVU is rarely used in children unless detailed anatomy of the calyces or ureter is required.

12.1 How long have you had the headaches?

Do they come and go, or are they continuously present?
Where are the headaches located?
How bad are the headaches? Do they stop you from doing things or
can you continue to do what you are doing? Are they getting worse or
are they much the same as when they first occurred?
Are there any associated features – e.g. nausea, vomiting, abdominal
pain and photophobia?
Are there any visual disturbances – e.g. loss of visual field, seeing odd
shapes and patterns (seeing zig-zag lines) or double vision?
Is there any altered sensation, e.g. pins and needles (parasthaesiae)
or weakness in any limb or limbs?
How is the headache relieved? Do you need to lie down in a quiet,
dark room to sleep? Is any medication being taken for relief and how
well does it work?
Does the headache get worse when lying down? Is it worse first thing
in the morning or any other time of the day?
Is there any family history of headaches or migraine?
How is school performance? Is there any concern regarding friends or
bullying?
Is there any parental discord?
Are there any triggers of the headaches – e.g. milk, cheese,
chocolates and eggs?

Discussion

Headaches are common in children and taking a detailed history is crucial in
their evaluation. Migraine and tension headaches are most common;
intracranial tumours, hypertension and pseudotumour cerebri must also be
considered in the differential diagnosis.

Migraine presents as episodes of pallor, vomiting, photophobia and
headaches followed by sleep and then recovery. These episodes are often
preceded by visual aura, bright spots/lines, flashes and blurred images, and
have recognized triggers. A family history is often present. The headache can
be one sided often with associated scalp tenderness. Migraine can be
complicated by paraesthesiae, difficulty in speech or hemiparesis –
hemiplegic migraine. Analgesics do provide some relief.

Tension headaches are more common in the older child and usually have
an associated life event, e.g. bullying at school, stress of school
examinations, domestic violence and parental disharmony.

Both of the above are intermittent. Intracranial tumour usually develops
gradually with continuous headaches which are characteristically worse first
thing in the morning (i.e. upon wakening) or upon lying down. It can,
however, present suddenly with a bleed into the tumour or with ataxia. Loss
of weight, nausea and vomiting and other neurological symptoms may be
present, e.g. diplopia.

Despite a detailed history and examination, it is often not possible to
differentiate between the above – an early referral for a CT scan (now widely
available) can be life saving!

13.1

A A large translucent area in the right side of the chest. The lung on this side is collapsed. The right hemidiaphragm is flattened. Except for the translucency extending to the left side, the left lung field appears homogeneously dense. An endotracheal tube is present.
Diagnosis – right tension pneumothorax.

B Enlarged cardiac shadow. Mild hyperinflation – the 8th rib is visible anteriorly.
Diagnosis – cardiomegaly.

C Sail-shaped opacity extending from the upper part of the mediastinum into the right lung field.
Diagnosis – thymus.

14.1 Hepatic cirrhosis with portal hypertension.

14.2 Hypersplenism.

14.3 d

Discussion
This girl has hepatic cirrhosis with portal hypertension – one of the commoner causes of cirrhosis in childhood. Among patients with cystic fibrosis the overall incidence of this complication is in the region of 5–10%. Hypersplenism explains the low white cell count, platelets and haemoglobin. Blood loss, e.g. bleeding varices and nutritional deficiencies, may also contribute to the low haemoglobin. Further investigations will include: a coagulation screen; an ultrasound scan of the liver and spleen; a liver biopsy to confirm and stage the severity of the cirrhosis and possibly an endoscopy to look for oesophageal varices.

15.1 Torsion of the testis and epididymitis.

15.2 Surgical exploration.

Discussion
Torsion of the testis occurs when the whole testis and epididymis twists on the spermatic cord, within the tunica vaginalis. It most often occurs around puberty and presents with acute abdominal pain radiating to the scrotum.

The scrotum and testes are swollen and tender to touch. Epididymitis is rare in childhood. Torsion of the hydatid of Morgagni is less severe and the history is not as acute as in torsion of the testis.

Most boys presenting with signs of torsion will require urgent surgical exploration; delay may result in avascular necrosis of the testes. At surgery the affected and normal testes are fixed in the scrotum.

| STATION 16 | ANSWERS | EXAM B |

16.1 a, d and f; c would also be accepted.

16.2 Janeway lesions. Osler's nodes and splinter haemorrhages.

16.3 Branch of right middle cerebral artery.

16.4 Infective endocarditis.

Discussion
This history suggests only one diagnosis – infective endocarditis. The most important investigation is a series of blood cultures which will help to identify the organism and its antibiotic sensitivity. A cardiac ECG should be done to identify and locate any vegetations or valve dysfunction. A cranial CT scan should be performed to document the nature of the cerebral lesion. Neurological examination suggests the intracranial lesion is in an area served by a branch of the right middle cerebral artery. Janeway lesions, splinter haemorrhages and Osler's nodes are all associated with infective endocarditis.

| STATION 17 | ANSWERS | EXAM B |

17.1 Exomphalos.

17.2 Cardiac, neurological or urological abnormalities.

17.3 See text.

Discussion
Exomphalos is the herniation of abdominal contents (mainly bowel, but can include liver, spleen and stomach) through the umbilical ring and into the umbilical cord. The hernia is covered by a transparent sac formed by the amniotic membrane and peritoneum. Associated congenital abnormalities affecting the cardiac, neurological and urological systems occur in up to 50% of cases. The diagnosis is usually made antenatally. After birth the abdomen is wrapped in several layers of cling film to minimize heat and fluid loss, and secretions aspirated via a nasogastric tube. Intravenous fluid replacement with dextrose or colloid, depending on the degree of fluid loss, is required. Smaller lesions can be surgically returned as a primary procedure; larger ones will require a gradual reduction.

18.1 a. true
    b. true
    c. true
    d. false
    e. true

Discussion
Following delivery, all newborns with breathing difficulties should be taken to a pre-warmed resuscitaire and actively dried with towels and then wrapped in a dry towel. Heat loss from wet skin quickly leads to a metabolic acidosis which will aggravate any apnoea. These measures take no more than a minute, at which time the baby's condition can be assessed and the 1-min Apgar mentally recorded. In an apnoeic baby the most important step is to establish ventilation. The baby's head should be slightly extended and with the facemask covering both the mouth and nose ventilation commenced at 40–60 per min using 100% oxygen. Most term babies will quickly respond and start breathing with these simple measures. Once respiration (and not before) has started naloxone can be safely given in cases where maternal opiate administration may be the cause of the apnoea. Oropharyngeal suction may induce a massive vagal outflow and induce apnoea and bradycardia. It is most likely when suction is aggressive. This child is not asphyxiated and does not require immediate intubation.

19.1 false

19.2 false

19.3 false

19.4 false

19.5 true

Discussion
G6PD and HS are the most likely diagnoses and are equally possible given the information. Spherocytes in a peripheral blood film are not diagnostic of HS as they may also be present in other blood disorders such as autoimmune haemolytic anaemias. Confirmation of HS requires the autohaemolysis test (increased rate of red cell fragmentation in isotonic solution). Increased fragility of HS red cells in hypotonic saline is also a feature. Splenomegaly and a positive family history (autosomal dominant) are also helpful diagnostic pointers. Pro-oxidant drugs promote haemolytic crises in G6PD. Parvovirus is well known to initiate aplastic crises in these three disorders.

20.1 d or e

20.2 d

20.3 f

20.4 a

20.5 b

20.6 c

Discussion

SMA – low birth weight is a cows' milk-based formula containing increased calories and protein to meet the increased requirements of low-birth-weight babies. Maxijul is a carbohydrate supplement added to milk to increase the energy content only; this is useful when total fluid requirements need to be restricted. Carobel is used to thicken feeds without increasing calories.

Pregestimil is a casein hydrolysate resulting in a semi-elemental diet that is lactose free and contains fat as medium chain triglycerides and protein as oligopeptides. It is easily digested and absorbed, reflecting a wide spectrum of usage: gastrointestinal immaturity or following surgery; severe idiopathic diarrhoea or lactose intolerance; cows' milk protein or other food allergy and transition from parenteral nutrition to normal diet. Wysoy is based on a soya protein and is also lactose free. Its uses include postgastroenteritis lactose intolerance and cows' milk protein allergy – however, it is normally used for this after the age of 1 year as soya allergy may develop.

Galactomin 17 does not contain galactose and is therefore useful in galactosaemia and galactokinase deficiency.

EXAM C

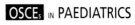

A 15-month-old toddler is investigated for poor appetite and failure to thrive. He was born at term weighing 3.8 kg (50th centile). His current weight is 8.2 kg (<3rd centile). He is an only child with no significant family history of note.

Investigations: Hb 8; serum iron – low, total iron binding capacity – decreased, serum ferritin – low.

Bone age 5 months.

The following statements are true or false:

1.1 A finding of a flattened villi on jejunal biopsy would confirm a diagnosis of coeliac disease.

1.2 A sweat sodium of 30 mmol/L is diagnostic of CF.

1.3 At least 50 mg of sweat needs to be collected before sweat sodium concentration can be used as a diagnostic marker for CF.

1.4 Hypothyroidism is a possible diagnosis.

1.5 The abnormal haematological indices exclude a diagnosis of emotional deprivation.

2.1 What is the diagnosis?

2.2 What are the two main presenting features after birth?

2.3 What complication may occur if not treated promptly?

2.4 What is the initial management?

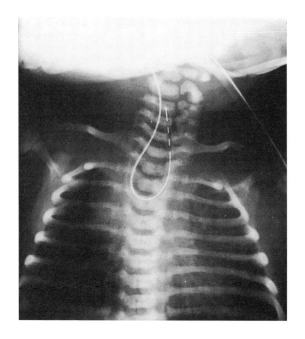

A 3-year-old boy is referred with a history of increasing puffiness and abdominal pain. He is noted to be miserable with a sallow complexion. Bilateral periorbital oedema is present and his hands and feet are cold. He has a distended abdomen but there is no guarding or tenderness. His axillary temperature is 37.1°C. Blood tests show Na 129 and urea 13.8.

3.1 What bedside test might help with the diagnosis?

3.2 Give the diagnosis.

3.3 Give two reasons which may account for the abdominal pain.

3.4 Why is the plasma sodium low?

3.5 Name two serious infections associated either with the disease or its treatment.

This child was systemically unwell with a fever.

4.1 What is the diagnosis?

4.2 Name two causes of this syndrome.

4.3 Other sites may be affected – choose the two most common from this list:
   a. conjunctiva
   b. meninges
   c. liver
   d. urethra
   e. kidneys.

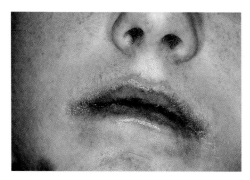

A

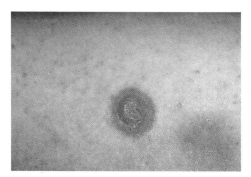

B

This picture is of a baby who presented at 7 days age with vomiting and weight loss. The birth weight was 3.0 kg; the weight now is 2.5 kg.

5.1 What is an acceptable degree of weight loss in the first few days of life?

5.2 Describe the abnormalities in this picture.

5.3 What is the diagnosis?

5.4 Name three serum biochemical abnormalities that may be present.

5.5 Name two tests that would help confirm the diagnosis.

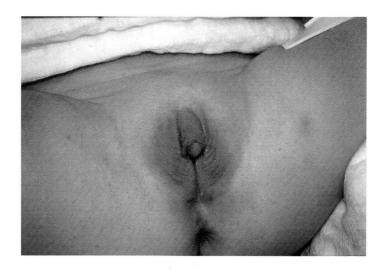

6.1   What are these lesions?

6.2   What is the most likely diagnosis?

6.3   What is the usual mode of inheritance?

6.4   Name one complication that can occur in each of the following systems:
- a. cardiovascular
- b. neurological
- c. orthopaedic
- d. ophthalmic.

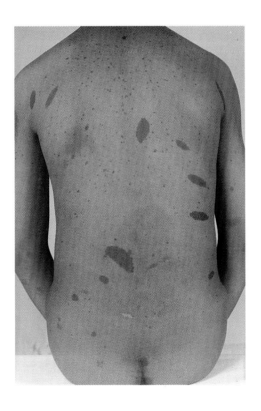

A 6-week-old, well baby, is diagnosed as having a ventricular septal defect (VSD) following an echocardiogram.

The parents ask the following questions:

7.1 Is our baby at any risk?

7.2 What is going to be the follow up, if any?

7.3 Should we be taking any special precautions?

7.4 Will he be able to run and play like other children?

7.5 What is the risk of the next child being affected?

Using short notes answer these questions.

A baby born at 37 weeks' gestation following a caesarean section presents with respiratory distress soon after birth with tachypnoea, recession and grunting. Although the baby is not requiring oxygen, an intravenous line is inserted to provide maintenance fluids. The mother had a temperature of 38°C and an offensive liquor before the birth.

8.1 Name three differential diagnoses.

8.2 What investigations should be carried out at this stage? Choose any number of the following:
a. blood culture
b. high vaginal swab from mother
c. blood sugar
d. microscopy of nasogastric aspirate
e. chest X-ray
f. serum urea and electrolytes.

8.3 What treatment would you institute at this stage?

9.1 Describe the features of the skin in these three patients and suggest a diagnosis for each.

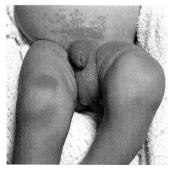

A

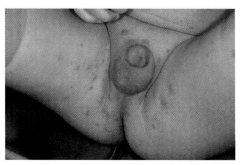

B

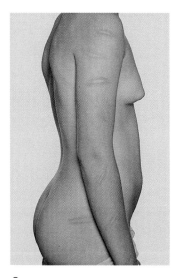

C

10.1 What investigation is shown in this slide?

10.2 Give three abnormal findings.

10.3 Give three long-term complications associated with this problem.

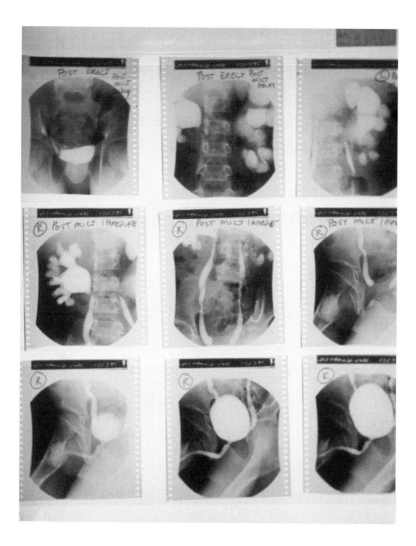

A 13-year-old girl with diabetes mellitus is admitted to hospital. Her sugar control had been good with glycosylated haemoglobin levels at no more than 1.0% above the normal range. However, since the beginning of this year and despite increases in insulin dosage there had been a marked deterioration in its control. She is in hospital for 48 h without a change in treatment, which consists of twice daily injections of a preparation containing short- and medium-acting insulin in a fixed ratio.

This is her glucose profile for the 48 h:

	day 1	day 2
pre breakfast	18	16
pre lunch	6	8
pre evening meal	14	12
midnight	2	3

Ketones are found in her urine on testing in the morning.

11.1 Give possible reasons for the deterioration in sugar control.

11.2 Explain the blood sugar results.

11.3 What adjustment to the insulin dosage needs to be made?

A 4-month-old baby is rushed to casualty because of laboured breathing. He was diagnosed as having bronchiolitis the previous day by his GP. On examination he is cyanosed, has shallow respiration at a rate of 10/min, is peripherally cold and is bradycardic with a heart rate of 30/min.

12.1 What is the immediate management? Choose one of the following:
   a. intravenous adrenaline and colloid
   b. nebulized salbutamol via oxygen
   c. ventilation with bag and mask or via an endotracheal tube
   d. cardiac massage
   e. intravenous atropine.

12.2 Despite your efforts above the baby has a cardiorespiratory arrest with the ECG monitor showing asystole. Name the two most useful drugs in this situation.

12.3 If intravenous cannulation was not possible, what alternative routes are recommended to give emergency drugs.

This girl presented with a sudden onset of facial asymmetry.

13.1 What is the neurological abnormality?

13.2 What is the most likely diagnosis?

13.3 Suggest two aspects of management.

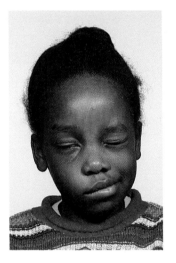 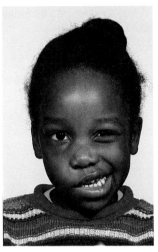

14.1 Describe the features on these X-rays and suggest a diagnosis for the first and the third.

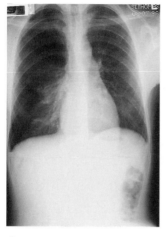

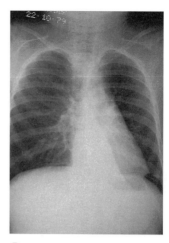

A   B

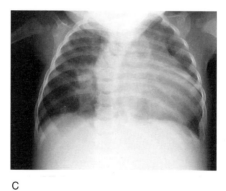

C

This is the CT scan of an 8-year-old boy 3 weeks after an episode of bacterial meningitis.

15.1 What is the main feature of this scan?

15.2 What is the diagnosis?

15.3 Which of the following are recognized complications of meningitis?
   a. subdural effusion
   b. deafness
   c. brain abscess
   d. cerebral palsy
   e. epilepsy.

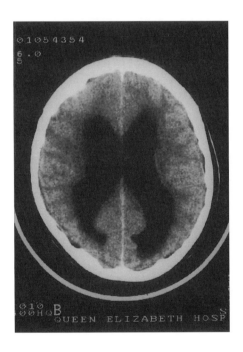

Michael, aged 5 years, has been noted to have been inattentive by his mother and teacher for the past six months. Initially, his GP thought that this may be due to poor hearing but the results of an audiology test were normal. He is seen by a paediatrician who finds a healthy boy with no evidence of developmental delay and notes that Michael himself is unaware of being inattentive. The paediatrician organizes one investigation with the result shown below.

16.1 What investigation is this?

16.2 Describe the result.

16.3 Which syndrome is indicated by the history and the result of the test?

16.4 How might his 'inattentiveness' be brought out during the test?

16.5 What two drugs are used in the treatment of this disorder?

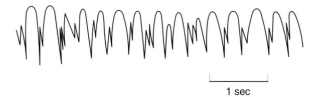

1 sec

A 9-year-old boy with sickle cell disease is admitted with severe abdominal pain.

On examination he is slightly jaundiced with a heart rate of 160/min, and there is a soft systolic murmur at the lower left sternal edge and aortic area; the apex is not displaced. There is no hepatosplenomegaly, but the abdomen is distended with generalized tenderness but no guarding.

Investigations: Hb 7, WCC 21, Plat 437, Na 144, K 5, Urea 6, Creat 113.

Answer 'true' or 'false'

17.1 Parenteral opiate analgesia is contraindicated.

17.2 Blood transfusion is required as there are signs of cardiac decompensation.

17.3 Intravenous fluids therapy should be instituted as dehydration predisposes to red cell 'sickling' in sickle cell patients.

17.4 The presence of the murmur suggests aortic valve stenosis.

17.5 Acute pancreatitis must be considered high in the differential diagnosis.

17.6 Patients with sickle cell disease have a renal concentrating defect.

This is a growth chart of a 3-month-old baby

18.1 What is the most likely diagnosis?

18.2 Give three underlying causes of this.

18.3 How could the diagnosis be confirmed?

18.4 Name two management options.

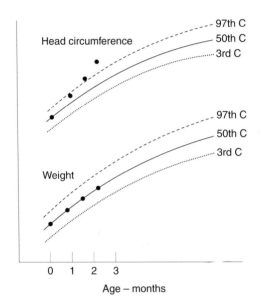

Match the clinical diagnosis (left-hand column) with the haematological finding most appropriate to it from the list in the right-hand column.

19.1 Kawasaki's disease   a.   Hydrops fetalis

19.2 Alpha-thalassaemia major   b.   Increased fetal haemoglobin

19.3 Beta-thalassaemia major   c.   Hyposplenism in a 6 year old

19.4 Sickle cell disease   d.   Oxidant-induced red cell damage

19.5 G6PD deficiency   e.   Splenomegaly in a 6 year old

19.6 Hereditary spherocytosis   f.   Thrombocytosis

The audiogram below is from a 5-year-old girl with learning difficulties. She was born at term and weighed 2 kg; Apgar scores 5 and 9 at 1 and 5 min respectively. She had several problems in the newborn period including a chest infection (treated with intravenous antibiotics), conjugated hyperbilirubinaemia and unexplained hepatomegaly with raised liver enzymes.

20.1 The threshold for hearing conversational speech is approximately:
    a. 0 decibels (db)
    b. 5 db
    c. 30 db
    d. 50 db.

20.2 The frequency range over which the human ear can detect sound is approximately:
    a. 100–500 Hz
    b. 100–1000 Hz
    c. 125–8000 Hz
    d. 0–500 Hz.

20.3 The audiogram indicates:
    a. bilateral high-frequency sensorineural hearing loss
    b. mixed conductive and sensorineural hearing loss
    c. bilateral conductive hearing loss
    d. bilateral low-frequency hearing loss.

20.4 The most likely cause for the hearing loss is:
    a. birth asphyxia
    b. neonatal hyperbilirubinaemia
    c. gentamicin toxicity
    d. Cytomegalovirus (CMV) embryopathy.

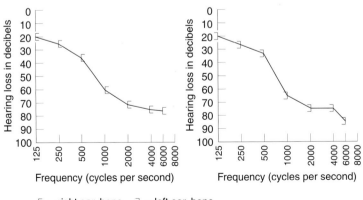

[– right ear, bone   ] – left ear, bone

The following questions relate to the karyotype shown.

21.1 Write down the karyotype and the associated syndrome.

21.2 What is the usual inheritance?

21.3 Which non-morphological clinical finding aids diagnosis in the newborn?

21.4 Give a common cardiac anomaly associated with this condition.

21.5 Give two reasons for speech delay.

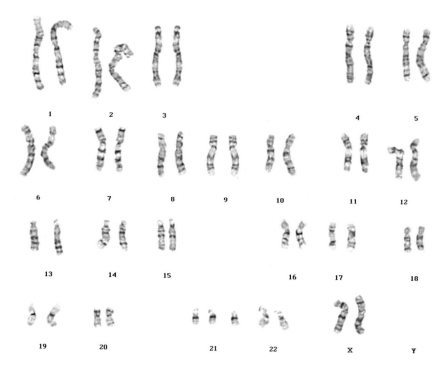

1.1 false

1.2 false

1.3 false

1.4 true

1.5 false

Discussion

There are several disorders associated with a picture of flattened villi on jejunal biopsy. A clinical response to a gluten-free diet in the presence of typical biopsy findings (hypoplastic villous atrophy) would be considered diagnostic of coeliac disease. Until recently, a post-treatment biopsy showing resolution of the atrophy and subsequent relapse following gluten challenge were also part of the diagnostic criteria. These criteria are now only used in atypical cases.

A sweat sodium of 60 mmol/L in a sweat sample weighing more than 100 mg is usually diagnostic of CF. The sweat chloride (>70 mmol/L) is also raised. Genetic tests are also helpful. The CF gene is on the short arm of chromosome 7. The gene codes for a cell membrane protein called the 'cystic fibrosis transmembrane regulator' which controls chloride and water movement in and out of the cell. The commonest single mutation is found at the delta-F 508 locus of the gene and involves deletion of this codon. In the homozygous state this mutation results in CF.

2.1 Oesophageal atresia.

2.2 Excessive oral secretions with episodes of coughing and choking or cyanosis.

2.3 Aspiration pneumonia.

2.4 Nasogastric suction and intravenous fluid replacement therapy.

Discussion

Oesophageal atresia has an incidence of 1 in 4000 births, and is frequently associated with (up to 50%) other congenital abnormalities. Maternal polyhydramnios may have been present during pregnancy. After birth X-ray confirmation of the passage of a nasogastric tube into the stomach excludes the diagnosis of oesophageal atresia. In the X-ray the tube is coiled in the upper third of the oesophagus. Excessive oral secretions associated with difficulty in breathing and cyanosis can develop. Aspiration pneumonia is a possible complication in infants who have been fed. Pending surgical correction the immediate management is to clear the oesophageal pouch of secretions by naso-oesophageal suction and maintain hydration with intravenous therapy.

3.1 A urine analysis test for protein such as an Albustix test will be strongly postive.

3.2 Nephrotic syndrome.

3.3 Peritonitis, hypovolaemia or renal vein thrombosis.

3.4 Dilutional hyponatraemia.

3.5 Streptococcal and varicella zoster infections.

Discussion

Nephrotic syndrome is characterized by severe hypoalbuminaemia. The loss of plasma oncotic pressure reduces the normal transudation of water from the venular end of capillaries and results in oedema and hypovolaemia. Visceral blood flow is compromised (one cause of abdominal pain – coeliac axis ischaemia) and stimulates compensatory aldosterone and antidiuretic hormone production. Water is retained in excess of salt and leads to dilutional hyponatraemia and increases oedema. Nephrotic patients also have an increased risk of infection, especially peritonitis due to *Streptococcus pneumoniae* and disseminated varicella as a result of steroid immunosuppression. The risk of arterial and venous thromboses is also increased.

4.1 Stevens–Johnson syndrome.

4.2 Antibiotics and viral infections.

4.3 a and d

Discussion

Stevens–Johnson syndrome is the bullous form of erythema multiforme involving mucous membranes and skin. Herpes simplex virus, mycoplasma infection and antibiotics, especially sulphonamides, are recognized aetiological factors; in most cases the cause is not known. Eye involvement (conjunctivitis, corneal ulceration and uveitis), stomatitis with ulceration, crusting and urethritis is common. Other features include fever, polyarthritis and diarrhoea.

Mortality is in the region of 5–10% and is due largely to dehydration and secondary bacterial or viral infection. Some patients develop recurrent attacks.

5.1 Loss of 10% of the birth weight is usually acceptable.

5.2 Enlarged clitoris and fusion of the labia.

5.3   Congenital adrenal hyperplasia.

5.4   Low sodium, potassium and glucose.

5.5   See discussion.

Discussion
Congenital adrenal hyperplasia is the commonest cause of ambiguous genitalia, occurring once every 10 000 births. The commonest type is due to a deficiency of the enzyme 21-hydroxylase, resulting in decreased production of cortisone and aldosterone but increased production of testosterone. These abnormalities explain the majority of the features:

- hyponatraemia
- hypokalaemia
- hypoglycaemia
- adrenal insufficiency
- virilization of the female – enlarged clitoris and fusion of the labia
- precocious genitalia in the male – not usually manifest at birth.

Diagnosis is confirmed by chromosomal analysis, ultrasound imaging of the internal genitalia and the adrenal glands and adrenal steroid measurement. Acute management involves intravenous electrolyte, dextrose and steroid therapy. Long-term management of females involves genitalia reconstruction and steroid therapy while carefully monitoring growth and skeletal maturity.

Newborn babies can lose 10% of their birth weight in the first few days of life; by day 10 after birth this has usually been regained.

STATION 6	ANSWERS	EXAM C

6.1   *Café au lait* spots

6.2   Neurofibromatosis or Von Recklinghausen's disease.

6.3   Autosomal dominant.

6.4   See text.

Discussion
Neurofibromatosis has an autosomal dominant inheritance with up to 50% of cases arising from new mutations. Skin manifestations include *café au lait* spots, axillary freckling and nodules. All of these are generally exaggerated at puberty. Two divisions of neurofibromatosis are generally accepted:

Type 1
Neurofibromatosis 1 is coded for on chromosome 17 and tends to result in neurofibromas appearing on the course of peripheral nerves. Complications often occur as a result of compression of adjacent structures by these tumours, e.g. of the renal artery causing stenosis leading to hypertension. Erosion of vertebral bodies can occur causing scoliosis. Uncommonly neurofibromas may undergo malignant change.

Type 2
Neurofibromatosis 2 is coded for on chromosome 22 and tends to manifest after puberty, in the central nervous system. Bilateral acoustic neuromas are the main lesions presenting with deafness and facial nerve palsy. Compression of the optic nerve can result in visual field disturbance. There may, however, be considerable overlap between the two types.

STATION 7 ANSWERS   EXAM C

7.1 The majority of VSDs have a good prognosis. Most defects close spontaneously in the first few years of life. After this period the prognosis is as good as for any other child. Some defects, which are usually larger, may lead to heart failure, requiring pharmacological treatment, and, if uncontrolled on this, surgery.

7.2 Approximately 10% are in this group.
The child is normally followed up in the clinic where an assessment of the defect involving clinical examination and an ECG ± an echocardiogram is carried out.

7.3 The only special precaution that the parents need to take involves prophylaxis against bacterial endocarditis. Bacteraemia from surgical procedures, including dental extractions, may result in the development of infected lesions – vegetations on the heart or heart valves. Antibiotic prophylaxis is therefore essential while these procedures are performed.

7.4 These children in general should be encouraged to be just as active as any other child. Parents should be dissuaded against overprotectiveness.

7.5 The recurrence risk for VSD and for congenital heart disease in general is approximately three times higher than normal, i.e. 5–6%.

STATION 8 ANSWERS   EXAM C

8.1 Gp B Strep pneumonia, transient tachypnoea of the newborn and hyaline membrane disease.

8.2 a, b, c, d and e

8.3 Antibiotics – penicillin at high dose and gentamicin.

Discussion
As *Group B streptococcal* pneumonia and sepsis are common and can be rapidly fatal, any newborn baby with respiratory distress must have this diagnosis considered. In this case with maternal pyrexia and an offensive liquor this is the most likely diagnosis. Other diagnoses to be considered include: transient tachypnoea of the newborn, hyaline membrane disease

OSCEs IN PAEDIATRICS

and meconium aspiration. The initial investigations should include: blood culture, CRP, full blood count (including white cell differential), skin swabs, microscopy culture and sensitivity of nasogastric aspirate, urine and cerebrospinal fluid, blood sugar, maternal high vaginal swab and, finally, chest X-ray. Serum urea and electrolytes in the first few hours after birth are unnecessary as they reflect only maternal values. High-dose penicillin and normal-dose gentamicin, both given intravenously, is a recommended combination.

STATION 9	ANSWERS	EXAM C

9.1   a. An erythematous rash affecting the napkin area with satellite lesions. Erythema on right knee from contact with floor.
Diagnosis – candida nappy rash.
     b. Erythematous vesiculopapular lesions around the nappy area.
Diagnosis – chicken pox.
     c. Six linear, 4–7-cm-long lines of pallor bordered by erythema on the arm, shoulder and buttock of a pubertal girl.
Diagnosis – non-accidental injury.

STATION 10	ANSWERS	EXAM C

10.1   Micturating cystourethrogram.

10.2   Bilateral dilated ureter, bilateral dilated renal pelves, blunted calyceal fornices, vesicoureteric reflux.

10.3   Recurrent urinary tract infections, renal failure and renovascular hypertension.

Discussion
This child has gross vesicoureteric reflux and is likely to suffer from recurrent urinary tract infections. Renal damage and scarring leading to renal failure and/or renovascular hypertension are likely long-term complications of recurrent UTIs. In the main, vesicoureteric reflux is managed with antibiotic prophylaxis. Surgical reimplantation of ureters would be considered in a child with gross reflux, as in this case.

STATION 11	ANSWERS	EXAM C

11.1   This loss of diabetic control at the beginning of the year is likely to be related to the onset of puberty, which is a time of relative insulin resistance, not to mention the changes in self-awareness and lifestyle associated with the pubertal growth spurt that are well known to affect control.

11.2   Somogyi effect.

11.3 The initial management of nocturnal hypoglycaemia is to decrease the evening insulin dosage.

Discussion

The blood glucose profile shows nocturnal hypoglycaemia in conjunction with early morning hyperglycaemia and ketonuria. This is characteristic of the *Somogyi effect* – excessive nighttime insulin levels leading to hypoglycaemia which stimulates counter-regulatory hormone secretion causing hyperglycaemia and ketonuria.

STATION 12	ANSWERS	EXAM C

12.1 c

12.2 Adrenaline and sodium bicarbonate

12.3 Intraosseous and endotracheal

Discussion

In an emergency situation in hospital there are usually a number of 'carers' who can perform a number of tasks. However, in this situation, where the baby is pre-terminal, all efforts must be directed to the respiratory system. This rule applies to all situations where the child is seriously ill and a number of the bodily systems are compromised. This baby should be ventilated, as a priority, with either bag and mask or via insertion of an endotracheal tube. Secondly, cardiac massage should also be given as the heart rate is inadequate. Salbutamol has largely no role to play in bronchiolitis, whether or not this is associated with cardiorespiratory compromise.

During a cardiac arrest with asystole in children the most useful drugs to give include adrenaline (inotrope and chronotope), sodium bicarbonate (for metabolic acidosis) and colloid (to improve the circulating volume).

Peripheral venous cannulation is frequently not possible in these situations. Intraosseus cannulation at the upper end of the tibia or the lower end of the femur is very likely to be effective in this age group. Adrenaline can also be given by the endotracheal tube.

STATION 13	ANSWERS	EXAM C

13.1 Lower motor neurone lesion of the right VIIth cranial nerve.

13.2 Bell palsy.

13.3 Oral steroids and eye protection.

Discussion

This girl has facial weakness of the whole of the right side of the face due to a lower motor neurone lesion of the VIIth cranial nerve – Bell palsy. The aetiology of this is unclear although it is probably post-infectious; herpes simplex virus infection is particularly implicated. Cranial fossa tumours (CT scanning may be required to exclude this), hypertension, sarcoidosis and Guillain–Barré syndrome need to be considered in the differential diagnosis. The early use of corticosteroids may hasten recovery which usually takes weeks but sometimes months. Eye protection with hypermellose eye drops and an eye patch are usually required overnight to prevent corneal ulceration and conjunctivitis.

| STATION 14 | ANSWERS | EXAM C |

14.1 a. Collapse of right lung. Increased translucency of the pleural space outside the right lung field.
Diagnosis – right pneumothorax.

    b. This rotated chest X-ray shows a hemivertebra between T6 and T7. The lung fields show hyperinflation with flattening of the diaphragms. Bilateral perihilar shadowing is present. There is cardiomegaly – this is, however, difficult to interpret in a rotated film.

    c. The left oblique fissure is displaced medially showing as an oblique line extending from the centre of the mediastinum to the left diaphragm behind the heart shadow. There is loss of the diaphragmatic shadow adjacent to this oblique fissure. The left lung field not superimposed by the heart shadow is more translucent compared to the right.
Diagnosis – left lower lobe collapse.

| STATION 15 | ANSWERS | EXAM C |

15.1 Dilated lateral ventricles.

15.2 Hydrocephalus.

15.3 a, b, c, d, e

Discussion
This scan shows dilated lateral ventricles – a feature of hydrocephalus. Following meningitis, this is thought to be a result of impaired resorption of cerebrospinal fluid (CSF). Cerebral abscesses manifest as space-occupying lesions with their associated signs, and a fluctuating temperature. Local cerebral infarction can result in subsequent epilepsy or in the development of cerebral palsy. Subdural effusion – often associated with *Haemophilus influenzae* meningitis – usually resolves spontaneously. Cranial nerve paresis, especially of the VIIIth nerve, can occur, resulting in deafness. All children after an episode of bacterial meningitis should have an audiological assessment at follow up.

16.1 An electroencephalogram.

16.2 3 per second 'spike and wave activity'.

16.3 Petit mal epilepsy.

16.4 Hyperventilation.

16.5 Sodium valproate, ethosuximide.

Discussion
Michael's history is typical of a child who has developed idiopathic generalized absence epilepsy or petit mal. The differential diagnosis is complex partial epilepsy (temporal lobe epilepsy – TLE) which is normally associated with various types of sensory aura. Petit mal has a much better prognosis – nearly all children will stop by early adolescence. Treatment is specific and different to TLE; sodium valproate and ethosuximide are the drugs of choice. Hyperventilation is used as a provocation test to induce epileptiform phenomena.

| **STATION 17** | ANSWERS | **EXAM C** |

17.1 false

17.2 false

17.3 true

17.4 false

17.5 false

17.6 true

Discussion
Effective analgesia is mandatory in the management of a severe crisis in patients with sickle cell disease. Intravenous opiate infusion is the most effective means of achieving this. This child has a 'visceral crisis', which is a common problem in childhood sickle patients, and he is dehydrated, which is likely to further promote sickling. Intravenous hydration is therefore indicated. The slight jaundice suggests that there is some degree of haemolysis, but a haemoglobin of 7 is not uncommon in well patients. In this boy the real haemoglobin may in fact be lower due to haemoconcentration. Cardiac 'flow murmurs' are often present in sickle cell patients and the tachycardia is a result of many factors, including pain. Neither of these findings per se indicate cardiac decompensation and he does not require blood transfusion based on these findings. There is a renal concentrating defect due to infarction of the vasa recta and this further increases the risk of dehydration. There is no tendency to develop aortic stenosis.

18.1 Hydrocephalus.

18.2 Intracranial haemorrhage, aqueduct stenosis and meningitis.

18.3 Cranial US or CT scanning.

18.4 Ventricular shunt or serial CSF taps.

Discussion

This growth chart showing rapidly increasing head circumference with normal growth along the weight centiles is most likely to be due to hydrocephalus. In familial large head the head circumference, although increased, remains parallel to the weight centile. Causes of hydrocephalus include intracranial haemorrhage, intracranial infection, aqueduct stenosis, Arnold–Chiari malformation and vascular malformations. The diagnosis can be confirmed by US scan, CT scan or magnetic resonance imaging (MRI) of the head. Management depends on the cause; most children will however require insertion of a ventricular shunt. In certain circumstances, serial CSF fluid taps may halt the progress of hydrocephalus prior to shunting.

19.1 f

19.2 a

19.3 b

19.4 c

19.5 d

19.6 e

Discussion

Thrombocytosis is a feature of Kawasaki's disease but does not usually manifest until the second week following the onset of symptoms. In conjunction with coronary arteritis, the very high platelet count predisposes to the ischaemic heart disease associated with this childhood vasculitis syndrome.

Fetal haemoglobin tetramers consist of two alpha and two gamma chains, whereas two alpha and two beta chains form adult haemoglobin. Complete absence of a chain production leads to a severe fetal anaemia, hydrops fetalis, and is incompatible with life. Accordingly, beta-thalassaemia major presents in the first year of life and is associated with increased fetal haemoglobin production – a feature of many congenital chronic haemolytic anaemias.

Hyposplenism in sickle cell disease results from repeated splenic infarctions in early childhood (autosplenectomy). Like all patients without functional splenic tissue children with sickle cell disease are prone to pneumococcal infections and thus receive pneumococcal vaccination and penicillin prophylaxis.

G6PD deficiency may manifest in the neonatal period with a haemolytic anaemia and severe jaundice without any precipitating factors. In later life intercurrent illness or, more commonly, exposure to pro-oxidant drugs may induce haemolytic crises.

In the absence of a family history isolated splenomegaly and pallor may be the only features of hereditary spherocytosis.

STATION 20	ANSWERS	EXAM C

20.1 c

20.2 c

20.3 a

20.4 d

Discussion
The acquisition of normal speech and language relies on being able to hear. Speech may still be acquired by a child with hearing loss but learning will be affected where the loss is greater than 30 db – the threshold for hearing conversational voice. Most of the acoustic energy in speech falls between 500 and 2000 Hz but the human ear is capable of hearing across a wide range of frequencies (125–8000 Hz).

This girl has bilateral high-frequency sensorineural hearing loss as a result of congenital CMV infection. The history is not consistent with birth asphyxia (normal Apgar scores) or kernicterus (she had a *conjugated* hyperbilirubinaemia). Gentamicin toxicity is a possible diagnosis but does not fit with other aspects of the history, such as the hepatitis and low birth weight which point to an intrauterine problem. Rubella embryopathy is also a possible diagnosis.

STATION 21	ANSWERS	EXAM C

21.1 47 XX, a girl with Down syndrome (trisomy 21 also acceptable).

21.2 Sporadic.

21.3 Hypotonia.

21.4 Atrioventricular septal defect, ventricular septal defect, Fallot's tetrad.

21.5 Global developmental delay, sensorineural and conductive hearing loss or hypothyroidism.

OSCEs IN PAEDIATRICS

Discussion

Most parents of a child with Down syndrome have a normal karyotype; the inheritance is sporadic and results from non-dysjunction of sister chromosomes (21) during gametogenesis (recurrence risk ~1%). Importantly, 10% of children with trisomy 21 have one parent with a balanced translocation (usually chromosome 21 attached to chromosome 11). The recurrence risk for such couples is much higher (~10% if mother carrier, ~2% if father carrier). Down syndrome can occasionally be a difficult diagnosis to make, especially in the newborn. Some common features all doctors should know include: mongoloid slant to eyes, low-set ears, incurving of the little fingers (clinodactyly), flattening of the occiput (brachycephaly), single palmar creases and increase in the space between the first and second toes. Truncal and limb hypotonia is a consistent finding that aids diagnosis in equivocal cases. The number of associations with trisomy 21 are legion and include: congenital heart defects (commonly atrioventricular septal, ventricular septal defects and Fallot's tetralogy (other structural defects are less common); GI tract problems (intestinal atresias, Hirschprung's disease, constipation); eyes, cataracts and short-sightedness; ears, sensorineural deafness, chronic otitis media leading to conductive hearing loss; CNS, moderate to severe global developmental delay (avoid the phrase 'mental retardation'), Alzheimer's type dementia manifesting after the age of forty. The incidence of childhood leukaemia and hypothyroidism is also increased. Fallot's tetralogy includes: ventricular septal defect, pulmonary stenosis, right ventricular hypertrophy and overriding of aorta.

EXAM D

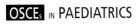

John, a 3-week-old infant, is found to be unwell in the special care baby unit. Born at 31 weeks' gestation with a birth weight of 900 g (<3rd centile), he developed respiratory distress syndrome within hours of birth. He was treated with surfactant therapy and mechanical ventilation. 12 days after birth he was extubated and on day 15 started milk feeds via a nasogastric tube. Over the last few hours he has become intolerant of his feeds.

On examination he is pale and jaundiced with a temperature of 35°C. Respiratory rate 50/min with mild recession. Heart rate 160/min. Marked abdominal distension is present with bile being aspirated via the nasogastric tube.

Investigations: arterial pH 7.14, P_{CO_2} 4.9 kPa, P_{O_2} 6.6 kPa, base excess (BE) 19 mmol, Hb 8, WCC 2, Plat 65.

1.1 The blood gas results indicate:
     a. a mixed respiratory and metabolic acidosis
     b. a compensated respiratory acidosis
     c. a metabolic acidosis
     d. an uncompensated respiratory acidosis.

1.2 The most likely finding on auscultation of the abdomen is:
     a. an absence of bowel sounds consistent with an ileus
     b. excessive bowel sounds consistent with an ileus
     c. normal bowel sounds
     d. excessive bowel sounds indicative of small bowel obstruction.

1.3 The most likely explanation for the blood results is:
     a. occult bleeding
     b. bone marrow failure secondary to severe sepsis
     c. disseminated intravascular coagulopathy
     d. a combination of a, b and c.

1.4 What is the most likely diagnosis?

John, aged 13 years, had surgery for a complex congenital heart lesion 3 weeks ago and is found to have a slow heart rate. This is his ECG.

2.1   What is the atrial rate?

2.2   What is the ventricular rate?

2.3   What is John's ECG diagnosis?

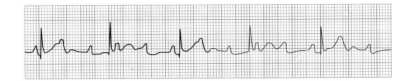

This X-ray is from a boy with a painful leg and a temperature of 37.8°C.

3.1   What are the abnormalities on the X-ray?

3.2   What is the diagnosis?

3.3   What investigation, not involving the taking of blood, could help confirm the diagnosis?

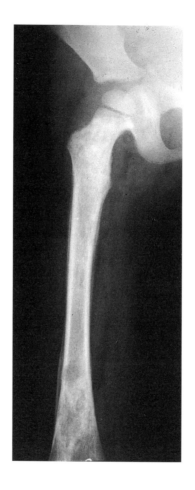

4.1 What is the pattern of inheritance illustrated in this family tree?

4.2 Give a clinical example?

4.3 What is the likely risk of disease manifestation in the children of the proband? Choose one of the following:

    a. none
    b. 1 in 2
    c. 1 in 4
    d. 1 in 8.

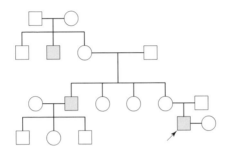

Michael, aged 18 months, is brought to his GP as his parents are worried that he may have developed epilepsy. They have noted that over the past 2–3 weeks he has sudden attacks of loss of consciousness. These episodes are preceded by him crying angrily for a couple of minutes and then turning blue. There are no abnormal limb movements and after a minute or so he gets up without any residual problem. His development has been normal and there is no family history of note. Physical examination is unremarkable.

5.1 What is the most likely diagnosis?

5.2 Which investigations would you perform at this stage? Choose any of the following:
a. CT scan of head
b. skull X-ray
c. EEG
d. ECG
e. blood sugar
f. none of these.

5.3 What is the management?

A 5-year-old boy has been rushed into casualty, having become unconscious while playing football at school. On examination he is responsive to pain but there is no evidence of trauma. His blood pressure is 170/110 and his pulse rate 70/min. Respiration is depressed. There is neck stiffness and absence of tendon reflexes. This is the finding on fundoscopy.

6.1 What does the picture show?

6.2 What is the most likely diagnosis?

6.3 What investigation is contraindicated?

6.4 What life-threatening complication is he at risk of developing?

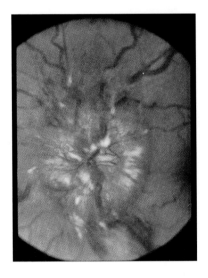

7.1 Describe the features on each of these X-rays and suggest a diagnosis.

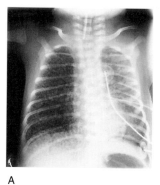

A

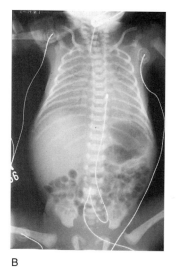

B

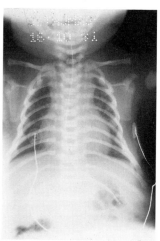

C

A previously well 2-year-old girl is brought to her GP with a 24-h history of fever and poor appetite.

On examination she has a slightly red throat. A throat swab is taken and the mother given a urine bag and asked to return the specimen when passed. Two days later the child is brought back to the GP with a persistent fever but her mother feels she is getting better.

The GP notes that the throat swab result has not returned but the urine culture shows a growth of three different organisms including *Staphylococcus epidermidis*. There were no WCC/RBC on microscopy.

8.1   What is the most likely explanation for the urine result?

8.2   What should the GP now do? Choose from the following:

     a. treat with oral antibiotics for 1 week

     b. treat with oral antibiotics for 2 weeks

     c. treat with oral antibiotics for 1 week and then arrange a DMSA scan and renal ultrasound

     d. repeat the urine culture

     e. arrange for a suprapubic aspiration of urine.

This rash developed spontaneously in a 2-year-old girl who was systemically well with no pyrexia.

9.1 What are the differential diagnoses?

9.2 Which is the most likely diagnosis?

9.3 What is the most important initial investigation?

9.4 What is the prognosis of your chosen diagnosis? Choose one of the following:
   a. 10% mortality
   b. 85% spontaneously recovering by 6 months
   c. 80% mortality
   d. 20% spontaneously recovering by 3 months.

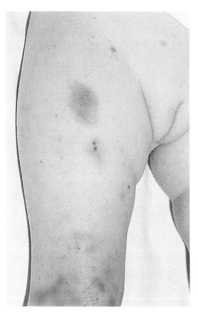
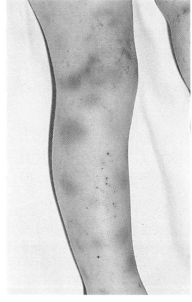

The girl in these pictures has a height below the third centile. The blood pressure in the right arm is 140/100 and in the right leg is 70/40.

10.1 Name three abnormalities present in the pictures.

10.2 What is the most likely diagnosis?

10.3 What investigation could confirm the diagnosis?

10.4 What is the likely cardiac diagnosis?

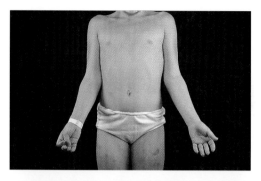

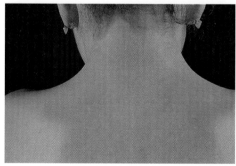

A 2-year-old boy is brought to the GP as his parents are concerned about him eating non-food items. His mother has found him eating paper, dirt from the garden and also strands of wool fibres from his clothing.

On examination the GP notes that he is below the third centile for height and weight.

11.1 Give three possible causes for these findings.

11.2 Explain how each of the diagnostic possibilities might be evaluated.

This girl presented with a painful right eye.

12.1 What is the diagnosis?

12.2 What complications can occur? Name three.

12.3 Name one microbe that may cause this.

12.4 What is the treatment of choice? Choose one of the following:
   a. oral flucloxacillin
   b. IV flucloxacillin and amoxycillin
   c. IV ceftazidime
   d. oral cefaclor
   e. IV gentamicin.

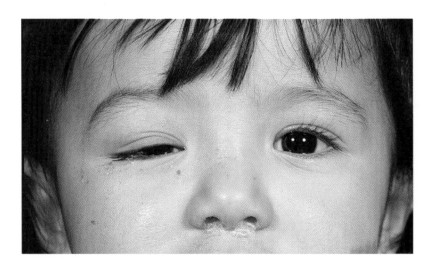

A 7-year-old boy with asthma is referred to the clinic for assessment. He has been on beclomethasone dipropionate 100 μg b.d. and salbutamol 100 μg p.r.n. via aerosol and spacer device for the last year. When questioned about the severity of the asthma, the boy replied, 'It's not too bad'.

13.1　What history might help you objectively gauge the severity of his asthma?

13.2　The history and examination lead you to suspect that his asthma is chronically undercontrolled despite satisfactory compliance. Which of the following options would you consider as appropriate changes in management at this stage?
a. starting oral theophylline
b. increase dose of beclamethasone to 200 μg b.d.
c. start regular home nebulized beta-2 agonist therapy
d. start regular sodium cromoglycate therapy
e. change from aerosol and spacer device to a powdered inhaler
f. start inhaled long-acting beta-2 agonist
g. start low-dose regular oral steroids.

13.3　How might this boy's asthma be more objectively assessed in the future?

This is an MRI scan of a 12-year-old boy who presented with ataxia and headaches.

14.1 What is the diagnosis?

14.2 Where is the lesion?

14.3 Which of the following features, if present, would be consistent with the diagnosis?
   a. nystagmus
   b. bitemporal homonymous hemianopia
   c. rombergism
   d. dysdiadochokinesis
   e. dysarthria
   f. arreflexia of the left knee tendon reflex.

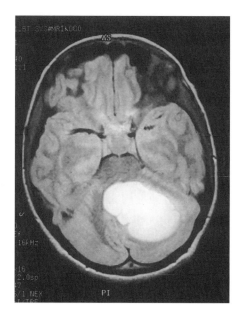

A 2-year-old boy is witnessed to have been unconscious for about 1 min following a head injury. Although he is fully alert now there is bruising on the left side of the head over the parietal bone. Skull X-rays are performed and he is admitted for neurological observations.

15.1 The presence or development of which of the following features would indicate the need for neurosurgical opinion and/or CT scanning?
   a. deteriorating level of consciousness
   b. a linear 5-cm-length fracture on the left parietal bone
   c. an increase in size of the left pupil with sluggish direct pupillary reflex
   d. a basal skull fracture
   e. seizures
   f. a decrease in blood pressure
   g. an increase in pulse rate.

15.2 What non-surgical, temporary manoeuvres can be performed to reduce raised intracranial pressure?

15.3 What advice needs to be given to the parents if by 24 h after admission the child has remained well and is ready for discharge?

A 2-year-old boy is brought in fitting for the last 25 min. He is placed in the recovery position and given facemask oxygen. Rectal diazepam is administered.

16.1 While waiting to see whether diazepam stops the fitting, what two bedside tests should you perform?

The following are three case histories:

A A 3-month-old infant was brought for his second DTP+Polio+Hib immunization. He has a runny nose and a slight cough but is generally well, apyrexial and feeding normally.

B A 4-month-old infant is brought to the surgery for his last DTP+Polio+Hib immunization. Following the previous immunization he developed erythema and a painful swelling affecting just over a quarter of the circumference of the upper arm around the site of the DTP injection.

C An 11-month-old infant is brought for the MMR immunization. He has diarrhoea and a temperature of 37.8°C.

17.1 Which infant(s) should have the immunization(s) postponed?

This is the growth chart of Fiona, who was born at term weighing 3.6 kg. She was breast fed for 4$^1/_2$ months with solids introduced at approximately 5 months of age. At 8 months of age she was referred to the hospital with a 3-month history of poor weight gain, intermittent diarrhoea and irritability.

On examination, she is pale with abdominal distension and mild wasting is noted, especially around the buttocks.

Investigations: Hb 9; WCC 9; Plat 430; Na 137, K 5.3, Urea 6.6, Ca 1.9, Albumin 35. Sweat test – normal.

18.1 What is the most likely diagnosis?

18.2 What investigation would confirm the diagnosis?

18.3 What treatment was instituted at 9 months of age?

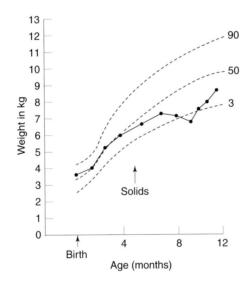

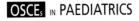

An 8-month-old infant is sent to casualty via his GP. The GP diagnoses 'wheezy bronchitis' but also notes that the child is unkempt, thin and has bruising on his back and forehead. He telephones you, the admitting paediatrician, explaining that there are serious concerns regarding non-accidental injury (NAI).

On examination there are no other signs of injury apart from the bruising mentioned. A chest X-ray shows mild bilateral hyperinflation and three rib fractures.

19.1   What is the most appropriate further management? Choose one of the following:

     a. admit the infant, inform parents of findings and then refer to a child psychologist

     b. admit the infant, do not inform the parents of findings relating to NAI but inform duty social workers

     c. admit the infant, inform the parents of findings and also the duty social workers

     d. allow infant home; request social workers and GP to follow up the case in the community

     e. admit the infant, inform social workers and request an emergency protection order.

19.2   Name three further investigations that are most useful at this stage.

19.3   At a subsequent case conference it was decided to put the baby under a supervision order. What is this?

Answer true or false
With regards to infant nutrition

20.1 Bottle-fed infants put weight on at a faster rate than breast-fed infants.

20.2 Breast feeding protects infants against infectious disease.

20.3 Breast-fed infants spend less time in rapid eye movement (REM) sleep than bottle-fed infants.

20.4 Breast- and formula milk-fed infants have identical amino acid profiles.

20.5 Breast milk and formula milk contain identical quantities of polyunsaturated fatty acids.

20.6 Breast-fed infants have less risk of developing atopic eczema than bottle-fed infants.

1.1 c

1.2 a

1.3 d

1.4 Necrotizing enterocolitis.

Discussion

This child is clearly unwell, needing supportive therapy (intravenous fluid and possibly mechanical ventilation) and broad-spectrum antibiotics. The abdominal distension and feed intolerance may be due to an ileus but necrotizing enterocolitis (NEC) should be considered especially as the Pco_2 suggests normal respiratory function. NEC is common in low birth weight infants and the initial signs are very subtle. However, the infant's condition rapidly deteriorates with signs of severe sepsis becoming more evident. Intestinal perforation may also occur during this early stage. Surgical referral may be necessary but most infants are managed conservatively. Plain abdominal X-ray films may show dilated loops of gas-filled bowel, air in the bowel wall (tramline appearance) or free air in the peritoneal cavity.

2.1 Atrial rate 70/min.

2.2 Ventricular rate 40 beats/min.

2.3 Third degree heart or complete heart block.

Discussion

A delay in or an absence of a QRS deflection following a P wave is by definition a form of heart block. An abnormally long interval between a P wave and a QRS complex describes first degree heart block. Second degree block describes the situation where only some P waves are conducted to the ventricles, invariably in a fixed ratio. If P waves fail to initiate QRS complexes at all, as in this case, complete or third degree heart block ensues. In children third degree heart block may be secondary to repair of complex congenital cardiac lesions. It may also be found in newborn infants with a structurally normal heart associated with maternal anti Rho/La autoantibodies in pregnancies complicated by systemic lupus erythematosus. Children with complete heart block are at risk of asystole and sudden death. Permanent pacemakers are the treatment of choice.

3.1 Periosteal reaction and hypodense areas adjacent to the metaphysis.

OSCEs IN PAEDIATRICS

3.2 Osteomyelitis.

3.3 Radionuclide bone scanning.

Discussion

Osteomyelitis and septic arthritis should be considered in the differential diagnosis in any child presenting with a painful limb and fever. This X-ray shows a periosteal reaction along the shaft of the femur with hypodense areas adjacent to the metaphysis. These findings strongly suggest a diagnosis of osteomyelitis. The X-ray features, seen here, usually take 7–10 days to develop. Radionuclide bone scanning will detect a septic focus (showing up as 'hot spots') much earlier. Blood cultures are mandatory and usually positive. Most infections are caused by *Staph. aureus*; other pathogens include *Strep. pneumoniae* and *Haemophilus influenzae*. *Salmonella typhimurium* needs to be considered in patients with sickle cell disease.

A periosteal reaction may be seen in a number of other disorders including bone tumours, trauma (including non-accidental injury (NAI)) and vitamin C and D deficiency.

STATION 4	ANSWERS	EXAM D

4.1 X-linked recessive inheritance.

4.2 Duchenne muscular dystrophy.

4.3 a

Discussion

In X-linked recessive inheritance associated with disease, the gene product of the 'normal' allele on one X chromosome prevents expression of the disease in a carrier female. In an affected male, there is no 'normal' allele counterpart on the Y chromosome. The gene product of the 'abnormal' allele on the X chromosome results in disease. In this form of inheritance females are only rarely affected, e.g. a carrier female marries an affected male; males cannot be carriers. Carrier females can show very mild signs or biochemical features of the disease. All the daughters of the index case will be carriers and his sons will be normal. There is therefore no risk of disease in his children. Duchenne muscular dystrophy, haemophilia and glucose-6-phosphate dehydrogenase deficiency exhibit this form of inheritance.

STATION 5	ANSWERS	EXAM D

5.1 Breath-holding attacks.

5.2 f

5.3 The best way of preventing these attacks is to avoid the child being provoked, although this is much easier to advise than to achieve. The other measure is to make as little fuss as possible when the child does have a breath-holding attack.

Discussion
Michael's parents give a history which is typical of breath-holding attacks. A normal cardiovascular examination and blood pressure are important negative findings. The parents should be reassured that the attacks are benign and hold no long-term implications despite their frightening nature.

STATION 6	ANSWERS	EXAM D

6.1 Papilloedema.

6.2 A subarachnoid haemorrhage/intracranial bleed.

6.3 Lumbar puncture.

6.4 Brainstem herniation/coning.

Discussion
The picture shows papilloedema. The history and examination suggest raised intracranial pressure and the most likely diagnosis is a large subarachnoid haemorrhage.

He is at risk of brainstem herniation and requires urgent transfer to a neurosurgical unit. Most importantly he needs a secure airway, which means he should be intubated and mechanically ventilated. A lumbar puncture is absolutely contraindicated.

STATION 7	ANSWERS	EXAM D

7.1 A Fine reticular shadowing of the right lung, left-sided chest drain, generalized opacity of the left compared to the right side of the lung, endotracheal tube and ECG leads.
Diagnosis: pulmonary interstitial emphysema with left-sided drained pneumothorax.

B Fine ground-glass appearance of both lungs, bilateral air bronchograms, umbilical arterial catheter, endotracheal tube and ECG leads.
Diagnosis: hyaline membrane disease.

C Reduced lung volumes bilaterally, bell-shaped chest, nasogastric tube and ECG leads.
Diagnosis: bilateral lung hypoplasia. Enlarged heart would receive some marks.

OSCEs in PAEDIATRICS

8.1   Contamination of urine with commensals.

8.2   d

Discussion
This a very common problem. A 'positive' urine result and a sick child. The temptation is to treat the child for a urinary tract infection. However, there were no white cells or organisms on microscopy and a positive growth of a skin commensal. The most likely explanation is that the culture result is due to contamination.

The child now needs to be examined to see if the cause of her fever is apparent and a repeat urine collection performed by someone with experience in collecting urine from toddlers. A child under 5 with a urinary tract infection needs further investigation which at a minimum includes an ultrasound scan. Hence, the importance of a definite diagnosis.

9.1   Meningococcal septicaemia, acute lymphoblastic leukaemia (ALL), non-accidental injury (NAI) and idiopathic thrombocytopenic purpura (ITP).

9.2   Idiopathic thrombocytopenic purpura.

9.3   Full blood count.

9.4   b

Discussion
Although ITP is the most likely diagnosis, meningococcal septicaemia, ALL and NAI should be considered in the differential diagnosis.

Meningococcal septicaemia is a rapidly progressive disease presenting with a sudden onset of malaise, fever and petechiae – drowsiness often does not occur until late into the illness.

ALL is marked by general malaise, pallor, lymphadenopathy and abdominal visceromegaly – usually developing over days if not weeks.

NAI is more likely if the above diagnoses are excluded and if there is a suggestive history, e.g. child is on the 'at-risk register', or other features on examination, e.g. bruising predominantly on the buttocks. Irrespective of the diagnosis, the most important initial investigation is a full blood count.

Some cases of ITP can be related to previous viral infections, e.g. rubella, or drug ingestion, e.g. co-trimoxazole. The commonest presenting features are spontaneous superficial bruising and petechiae; mucosal bleeding (nose bleeds) is uncommon. 85% have an acute self-limiting course and the majority have spontaneously recovered by 6 months. With platelet counts of less than 10 there is increasing risk of intracranial bleeding (extremely rare).

In difficult cases, bone marrow aspiration and trephine biopsy may need to be performed to exclude ALL.

Treatment is controversial and may include platelet infusions, steroids and intravenous immunoglobulins; most cases can be managed expectantly.

STATION 10	ANSWERS	EXAM D

10.1 Wide carrying angle (cubitus valgus), widely spaced nipples and webbing of the neck.

10.2 Turner syndrome.

10.3 Chromosomal analysis.

10.4 Coarctation of the aorta.

Discussion

This girl with a wide carrying angle (cubitus valgus), widely spaced nipples, neck webbing, a low hairline and short stature has Turner syndrome. The diagnosis can be confirmed by chromosomal analysis; in about 50% the 45 X0 karyotype is present. The others have either a deletion of one of the short arms of the X chromosome or one of a variety of other structural defects. Other features of Turner syndrome include: lymphoedema of hands and feet in the neonatal period, cardiac defects and ovarian dysgenesis resulting in infertility. In this case the cardiac diagnosis is most likely to be coarctation of the aorta. Intellectual development is normal. Aspects of management include growth hormone therapy and oestrogen replacement for development of secondary sexual characteristics during puberty.

STATION 11	ANSWERS	EXAM D

11.1 Neglect, iron deficiency anaemia and mental retardation.

11.2 Full blood count, a full developmental examination and a home assessment to exclude neglect.

Discussion

This boy has pica – the eating of non-nutritive substances. It is associated with various problems, including neglect, iron deficiency anaemia and mental retardation. He needs a full developmental examination, full blood count (FBC) and a home visit or health visitor assessment to exclude neglect. Note, all three conditions may coexist.

STATION 12	ANSWERS	EXAM D

12.1 Periorbital cellulitis.

12.2 Orbital cellulitis, cavernous sinus thrombosis, meningitis.

OSCEs IN PAEDIATRICS

12.3 *Staphylococcus aureus.*

12.4 b

Discussion

Periorbital cellulitis must be taken seriously and treated promptly as there is a significant risk of orbital cellulitis associated with proptosis, painful eye movements and reduced visual acuity, meningitis and cavernous sinus thrombosis. *Staph. aureus* and *Strep. pneumoniae* are most often implicated in its aetiology. *Haemophilus influenzae b* infection has now become rare as a result of the Hib vaccine. Out of the options listed, the best combination for treatment is therefore intravenous flucloxacillin and amoxycillin.

STATION 13	ANSWERS	**EXAM D**

13.1 See text.

13.2 b, d or e

13.3 Recording of peak expiratory flow rate (PEFR) and use of rescue medication in a diary card.

Discussion

The aim of asthma management is to minimize both daytime and nocturnal symptoms. The child should not miss nursery or school, participate fully in exercise or sports and should require relatively infrequent rescue therapy. Based on these aims an assessment of asthma severity can be made on the following information:

- Nocturnal symptoms. How often does asthma wake the child and parents during the night? How often does it prevent the child from going to sleep?
- School. How often does the child not go to school or gets sent home because of asthma?
- Exercise tolerance. Can the child keep up with his peers? How far can he run or walk before resting or needing treatment?
- Nebulizer therapy. How many GP or casualty visits have resulted in the need for nebulizer therapy?
- Steroid courses. How many GP or casualty visits have resulted in steroids being prescribed?
- Rescue therapy. How often is the beta-2 agonist therapy being used?

A number of therapeutic options are available to control symptoms under these circumstances. Out of those listed the following would be recommended. Increasing the dose of beclamethasone would perhaps be most beneficial. Although at present there is no evidence of significant side effects of steroids at this dose, some doctors and parents may prefer to use a second anti-inflammatory drug, in this case sodium cromoglycate, particularly if exercise-induced symptoms are prominent. Another option to consider is to change the form of inhalation from aerosol and spacer device to powdered inhalation. Starting theophylline, nebulized salbutamol, long-acting beta-2 agonist and low-dose oral steroid therapy would normally be saved for more severe cases where high-dose inhaled steroids and sodium cromoglycate have already been attempted.

Recording of the frequency of daytime and nocturnal use of rescue therapy and daily recording of peak flow rates would be useful in objectively assessing asthma severity in the future.

| STATION 14 | ANSWERS | EXAM D |

14.1 An intracranial mass/tumour.

14.2 Cerebellum – extending to the brainstem.

14.3 a, d, e

Discussion

The most common site for intracranial tumours in children is in the posterior fossa. The signs and symptoms are related to the development of raised intracranial pressure and dysfunction of the cerebellum. These are:

- Ataxia – broad-based gait, patient falters to side of lesion.
- Dysdiadochokinesis – slowness and incoordination of rapid alternating movements; supination followed by pronation of hands.
- Past pointing.
- Rebound overshoot.
- Coarse intention tremor – i.e. exacerbated by action.
- Nystagmus – a coarse horizontal nystagmus, worse when looking towards the side of the lesion.
- Dysarthria – a halting, jerking dysarthria, i.e. the scanning speech.
- Pendular reflexes – hypotonia and depression of reflexes are sometimes seen – not arreflexia – these can be slow or 'pendular'.
- Rombergism is a sign of sensory ataxia. Bitemporal homonymous hemianopia is a feature of lesions affecting the optic chiasma.

In this child the tumour, which was in fact an astrocytoma, can be easily seen as a dense mass projecting from the left side of the cerebellum towards and compressing the brainstem. The lesion compressed the CSF outflow tract, causing a severe obstructive hydrocephalus.

| STATION 15 | ANSWERS | EXAM D |

15.1 a, c, d and e

15.2 See text.

15.3 See text.

Discussion

Head injury following road traffic accidents and falls is the single most common cause of death in children in this country. Most head injuries are minor, although some children require admission for a short period of

OSCEs IN PAEDIATRICS

observation. At discharge, it must be stressed that if the child begins to vomit, becomes drowsy, has increasing headache, begins to fit, gets blurred or double vision, or is unwell in any other way then he must be seen by a doctor urgently.

The development or presence of the following would indicate the need for urgent neurosurgical opinion and/or CT scanning:

- Deteriorating level of consciousness, as assessed by the Glasgow or other recognized coma scale.
- Development of any focal neurological sign, e.g. abnormal pupillary size or reflexes and limb weakness.
- Seizures.
- Depressed or basal skull fracture. Uncomplicated linear fractures by themselves do not require further intervention.
- Increase in blood pressure and lowering of pulse rate. This is a late sign of raised intracranial pressure and implies impending coning. Decrease in blood pressure with increase in pulse rate is a feature of shock.
- Leakage of CSF through the nose or ear – implies a basal skull fracture.

Temporary manoeuvres that can be performed to reduce raised intracranial pressure include infusion of mannitol, artificial hyperventilation and nursing in a 30 degrees head-up position.

STATION 16	ANSWERS	EXAM D

16.1 Blood sugar and temperature.

Discussion
The initial management of a fitting child is important. After placing the child in a safe position oxygen should be administered. Thereafter, an initial dose of rectal diazepam will terminate the majority of fits. The next steps are to check the temperature and blood sugar – these are occasionally overlooked and will help in establishing the diagnosis and aid treatment. Those who fail to respond to diazepam need management as of status epilepticus.

This child will need careful examination and investigation. In febrile convulsion a source of infection should be sought; most commonly a viral illness is responsible, but more serious infections such as meningitis, pneumonia and pyelonephritis are sometimes found.

STATION 17	ANSWERS	EXAM D

17.1 Infant C.

Discussion
Parents should be offered to have their child immunized at every opportunity – in hospital or in the community. Careful consideration should be

undertaken before an immunization is delayed, and so an understanding of the general and specific contraindications to immunizations is important.
Contraindications include:

- The child is suffering from an acute illness, e.g. an upper respiratory tract infection or diarrhoea with fever and/or systemic upset.

Severe local or general reaction to previous immunization:

- Local. An extensive area of redness and swelling which becomes indurated and involves most of the anterolateral surface of the thigh or a major part of the circumference of the upper arm.
- General. Fever equal to or more than 39.5°C within 48 h of a vaccination; anaphylaxis; prolonged unresponsiveness or high-pitched, inconsolable screaming for more than 4 h; convulsions or encephalopathy occurring within 72 h.

In case A, where there is no fever or systemic upset, and in case B, where the local reaction was limited, the immunizations should not be postponed.

| **STATION 18** | ANSWERS | **EXAM D** |

18.1 Coeliac disease.

18.2 Jejunal biopsy.

18.3 Gluten-free diet.

Discussion
The onset of symptoms of diarrhoea and failure to gain weight (centile chart) with the introduction of solids strongly suggests coeliac disease (gluten-induced enteropathy). Giardiasis and cystic fibrosis also need to be considered in the differential diagnosis. The next investigation following a normal sweat test should be a jejunal biopsy. Antibodies to gliadin, reticulin and endomysium are commonly present in coeliac patients but are not diagnostic. The introduction of a gluten-free diet would account for the weight gain.

| **STATION 19** | ANSWERS | **EXAM D** |

19.1 c

19.2 Full blood count (FBC), skeletal survey and clotting screen.

19.3 See text.

Discussion
In all cases of NAI local child protection protocols should be followed. However, there are some procedures that are common to all. All cases of suspected or confirmed NAI of this severity need to be removed immediately from the environment where the harm is suspected to have taken place to a

place of safety, usually a hospital. If no medical treatment or further investigations are required, then placement in a children's or a foster home is more appropriate. The parents must be informed of the findings. If appropriately handled, i.e. without making any accusing remarks, most parents will accept hospital admission of their child for observation and further investigation. Occasionally this is not possible and legal enforcement in the form of an emergency protection order is required. Early involvement of social workers is essential; the at-risk register can be checked because siblings could be at risk and previous concerns regarding the family can be highlighted, etc.

The most useful investigations at this stage include FBC, clotting studies and a skeletal survey or a radioisotope bone scan.

Under a supervision order an infant or child returns to the family home but is kept supervised by a named person or authority. Extra conditions may be added: e.g. attendance at a specified place and time for medical or psychiatric treatment. It has a sanction in that failure to comply may result in the supervisor bringing the matter back to the court for alternative protection procedures to be implemented.

STATION 20	ANSWERS	EXAM D

20.1 true

20.2 true

20.3 true

20.4 false

20.5 false

20.6 true.

Discussion
Bottle-fed infants (cows' milk based feeds) do increase weight at a faster rate than breast-fed infants. This finding does not yet have any clinical associations. Breast feeding protects against infectious disease in both developed and developing countries. The time spent in REM sleep is thought to be an indicator of immaturity. There is increasing evidence that breast-fed infants have an increased rate of neurological maturation and hence this interesting finding. It is true to say that formula milk-fed infants have an abnormal plasma amino acid profile. There is no clinical evidence that this difference is detrimental to bottle-fed infants, although the availabilty or relative amounts of amino acids may be important in neurotransmitter formation. The quality of fat in breast milk is different to that in cows' milk-based feeds. The most important differences are related to essential fatty acids (EFA), which are important for central nervous system growth and development. Nerve growth (synapse formation and arborization) is critically dependent on the availability of these essential fatty acids and, until recently, commercial feeds contained no EFA supplementation.

EXAM E

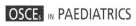

A 5-year-old girl is referred with an abdominal mass found by her mother as she was undressing her. She has had no significant medical problems in the past. On examination you note a mass arising from the right renal angle extending medially almost to the midline and inferiorly 10 cm. Her BP is noted to be 160/110.

Investigations: plasma urea, creatinine and electrolytes are normal; urine microscopy – haematuria +++; culture – no growth.

1.1 What are the two most likely diagnoses?

1.2 Explain why the blood pressure is raised in these two conditions?

1.3 For each diagnosis give one site where further lesions might be commonly found.

2.1 Describe the features and give the diagnosis for each of these X-rays.

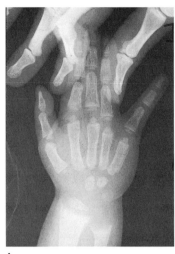

A

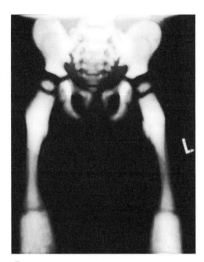

B

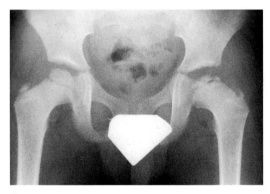

C

John, aged 3^1/$_2$ years, is seen by his GP because of continuing concerns about his development. He is the first child of unrelated parents and the pregnancy and birth were unremarkable. There is no family history of note. Presently, his mother is 12 weeks into the next pregnancy.

It is ascertained that John smiled at 3 weeks of age and was fixing and following at 1 month. He sat up alone at 10 months and started to crawl aged 1 year. By 18 months he was beginning to walk holding on to furniture, but he could not stand unsupported. He had minimal speech until 6 months ago but now can say 20–30 words with meaning. He is not yet dry by day. He is a happy boy and easy to look after.

In the clinic, it is noted that John walks with a distinct 'waddle'. He gets up from the floor by first rolling over onto his front and then pushing himself up.

3.1 What does the 'waddle' gait and the manner in which he gets up suggest?

3.2 What is this sign called?

3.3 Give the diagnosis and one confirmative test.

3.4 Why is it important to establish the diagnosis as soon as possible?

A 12-month-old infant is admitted with sudden difficulty in breathing, fever and cough following a few days of cold-like symptoms. On examination he has an obvious stridor and is tachypnoeic with moderate subcostal and intercostal recession. A loud barking cough is heard.

4.1 What is the diagnosis?

4.2 What is the usual aetiology?

4.3 Which of the following investigations would you carry out?
  a. throat swab
  b. X-ray of the upper airway
  c. viral titres
  d. laryngoscopy.

4.4 What is the initial management? Choose one of the following:
  a. rest in a comfortable environment with oxygen saturation monitoring
  b. 'a' and nebulized budesonide (Pulmicort)
  c. 'a' and regular nebulized ipratropium bromide (Atrovent)
  d. 'a' and regular nebulized adrenaline
  e. 'a' and intravenous antibiotics.

This 3-year-old child has been unwell for 3 days. Initially, his illness was felt to be caused by flu but over the last 24 h he has developed a rash and a painful left foot.

On examination he is unwell with a temperature of 38°C. Apart from this non-blanching rash, his left ankle is swollen and also tender on movement.

5.1 What does the slide show?

5.2 What other skin lesion is commonly associated with this syndrome?

5.3 What is the diagnosis?

5.4 Give one long-term complication.

5.5 Give one further clinical investigation that should be performed.

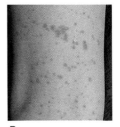

B

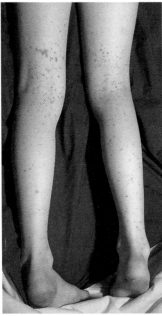

A

An 8-month-old infant is admitted with a 24-h history of persistent crying and going off his feeds. The crying is noted to be episodic and associated with leg and hip flexion. On abdominal examination a centrally placed 'sausage-shaped' mass is palpable.

6.1 What is the most likely diagnosis?

6.2 What may be found on rectal examination?

6.3 What investigations would you arrange at this stage? Choose one of the following:
a. plain abdominal X-ray and U&E
b. Contrast Gastrograffin enema and U&E
c. U&E, full blood count and abdominal ultrasound
d. U&E, urine for C&S and stool culture
e. U&E, FBC and abdominal CT scan.

6.4 What would be the diagnosis if, in addition to the above, the infant was lethargic and pale with abdominal tenderness and absent bowel sounds?

6.5 What would be the next two steps in management in order of priority?

Answer true or false to the following questions:

7.1 Neonatal mortality is the number of deaths per thousand live births within the first week of life.

7.2 Changes in neonatal mortality reflects standards of feto-maternal health and health care.

7.3 The data in the graph below suggest that the incidence of surfactant deficiency is decreasing.

7.4 Surfactant therapy causes bronchopulmonary dysplasia.

7.5 Increased survival because of surfactant therapy is the most likely reason for the increase in infants with bronchopulmonary dysplasia.

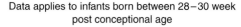

Data applies to infants born between 28–30 week post conceptional age

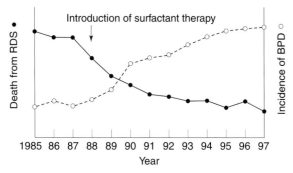

Match the inhalation device to the age group *most* likely to find the greatest benefit for the control of wheezing symptoms.

8.1 Volumatic.   Ages: 12 months

8.2 Babyhaler.   3 years

8.3 Turbohaler.   8 years

8.4 Metered dose inhaler.   15 years

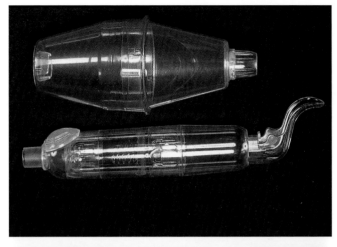

Volumatic

Babyhaler

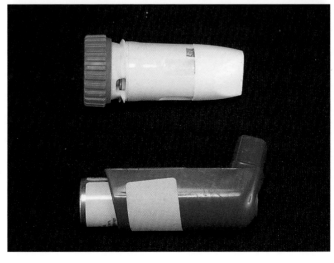

Turbohaler

Metered
dose inhaler

9.1 Give the diagnosis in each of these slides.

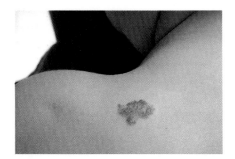

A

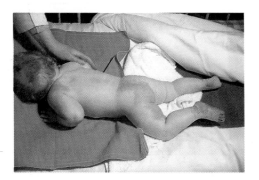

B

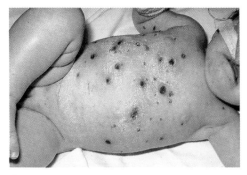

C

OSCEs IN PAEDIATRICS

A 4-week-old baby presents with a history of vomiting for 3 days. Despite the vomiting his mother reports that he is eager to feed. On examination he is dehydrated and apyrexial. Serum biochemistry shows:

sodium	128
potassium	3.0
chloride	86
urea	6.0
bicarbonate	36
pH	7.50

10.1 Describe these results.

10.2 Give three differential diagnoses.

10.3 What is the most likely diagnosis?

10.4 What further investigations should be carried out? Choose the three most useful from the following list:
a. differential white cell count
b. an oesophageal pH study
c. plain abdominal X-ray
d. urine for M,C&S
e. test feed
f. barium swallow.

11.1 What is the mode of inheritance shown in this pedigree?

11.2 Give two diseases showing this form of inheritance.

11.3 What is the risk of 'A' being a carrier?

11.4 What is the risk of an affected child if 'A' marries into the general population? Assume the carriage rate in the population is 1 in 40.

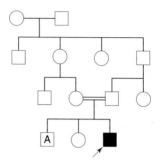

A six-week-old infant is referred for poor weight gain. On examination he looks cachexic and is dysmorphic with low-set ears and a very small lower jaw. He also has severe thrush affecting the oral cavity and perineum. The cardiac apex is displaced into the left sixth intercostal space, anterior axillary line, and there is a palpable thrill. A loud pan-systolic murmur and an apical mid-diastolic murmur can be heard. He is tachypnoeic but the lung fields are clear on auscultation. The liver is 3 cm below the costal margin in the midclavicular line.

Investigations: Na 136, K 4.9, Ca 1.7, albumin 42, Urea 7.8, Hb 10.2, WBC 3.8, Plat 245. Cardiac echocardiogram – large ventricular septal defect.

12.1 The diastolic murmur is caused by:
   a. tricuspid regurgitation
   b. mitral regurgitation
   c. increased blood flow across the mitral valve
   d. increased blood flow across the aortic valve.

12.2 The most likely explanation for the low plasma calcium is:
   a. fluid overload and is dilutional in origin
   b. that it is an artefact of venesection
   c. primary hypoparathyroidism
   d. intestinal malabsorption.

12.3 He is also found to have an immunodeficiency. This most likely results from:
   a. thymus gland aplasia/dysplasia leading to abnormal cell-mediated immunity
   b. splenic aplasia leading to abnormal handling of bacteria and fungal infections
   c. liver disease leading to combined defective T and B cell immunity
   d. thymus gland aplasia/dysplasia leading to defective humoral immunity.

12.4 This baby's features most likely result from:
   a. an embryological defect of the 3rd and 4th pharyngeal pouches
   b. trisomy 21
   c. rubella embryopathy
   d. HIV embryopathy and acquired immunodeficiency syndrome.

This is an X-ray of a 2-year-old boy who presented with difficulty in breathing, cough and a fever.

13.1 What are the features on this X-ray?

13.2 What is the diagnosis?

13.3 Name two non-antibiotic treatments which may be helpful.

13.4 Which one of the following is the most appropriate antibiotic regimen?
  a. cefadroxil
  b. penicillin
  c. flucloxacillin and ampicillin
  d. ciprofloxacin
  e. erythromycin.

13.5 What follow-up investigation is required?

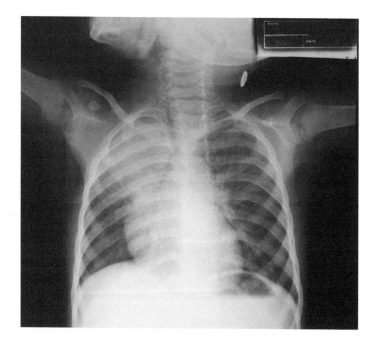

The parents of a 5-year-old boy come to see their GP as they are concerned that their son wets the bed. The GP takes a history and examines the boy.

14.1 What aspects of the history would point to a diagnosis of 'simple' nocturnal enuresis?

14.2 If the history and examination point to this diagnosis what, if any, investigation(s) should be performed?

14.3 What percentage of normal 5-year-old children have not reached bladder control at night?

Choose from the following:
a. 1%
b. 5%
c. 10%
d. 25%
e. 50%
f. other.

A 2-year-old girl is brought in with a history of fever, rash, neck stiffness and vomiting. A diagnosis of bacterial meningitis is suspected and a lumbar puncture is performed.

15.1 What three non-microbiological tests of the CSF would help aid the diagnosis?

15.2 Blood leaks into the CSF during the lumbar puncture. How does this affect your assessment of the tests in 15.1, and how would you compensate for this?

15.3 Microscopy confirms the presence of gram-negative diplococci. What is the most likely pathogen?

15.4 What is the most appropriate antibiotic therapy out of the following?
a. ceftriaxone
b. flucloxacillin and chloramphenicol
c. benzylpenicillin
d. benzylpenicillin and gentamicin
e. ceftazidime.

15.5 What prophylaxis should be considered?

16.1 What are the four development milestones shown in these pictures?

16.2 At what ages are these normally developed?

16.3 How old do you think this child is?

16.4 What is the expected speech development at this age?

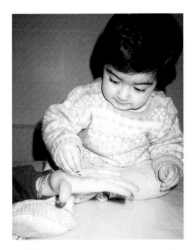

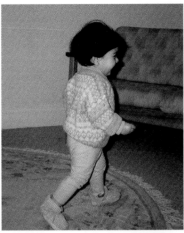

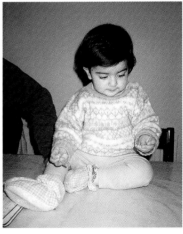

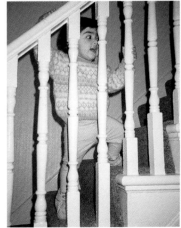

Fiona, aged 8 years, is admitted to hospital 3 weeks after a throat infection, having developed bilateral ankle pain and pain in her left hand over the last 4 days.

On examination she has a low-grade fever, and both ankles are swollen. She has pain on movement of the fingers of her left hand also with some swelling. No other joints appear to be affected and the rest of the physical examination is normal.

Four days after admission Fiona continues to have a fever. The pain in her ankles persists but there is now swelling of her right hand; her left hand is much better. A soft systolic heart murmur is present at the apex.

Investigations:

Hb 10, WCC 12, Plat 396. Serum electrolytes – normal.

Plain X-rays of hand and ankles – normal.

ESR days 1–34, days 4–65.

Blood cultures – negative.

Urine – no WCC or RBC and no organisms.

17.1 Give four investigations that might help to establish a diagnosis.

17.2 What is the most likely diagnosis?

This blood film and photograph of the palate is from a 12-year-old boy.

18.1 Describe the main features in each picture.

18.2 What is the diagnosis?

18.3 Give three complications that may occur.

18.4 What medication is contraindicated?

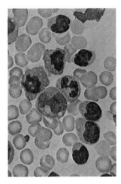
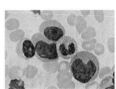
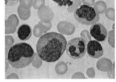
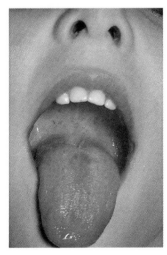

This question concerns the current national immunization schedule in the UK.

19.1 Fill in the name of the vaccine/s at the appropriate age group in the table.

Age	Vaccine/s
2 months	
3 months	
4 months	
12–18 months	
4–5 years	
10–14 years	
15–18 years	

Jane, a previously well 13-year-old, is brought into casualty with a sudden history of palpitations and shortness of breath. On examination she is sweating, slightly pale and anxious. Her pulse rate is noted to be above 200/min.

Her ECG is shown below.

20.1 What is the ventricular rate?

20.2 What is the ECG diagnosis?

20.3 How might you terminate this arrhythmia non-pharmacologically and how is this effect mediated?

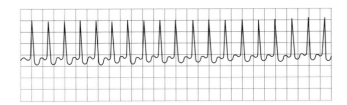

Concerning pulse oximetry.

21.1 Pulse oximeters measure
   a. the percentage of haemoglobin which is oxygenated
   b. the oxygen content of blood
   c. the partial pressure of oxygen
   d. the transcutaneous oxygen content of blood.

21.2 A 6-week-old infant with bronchopulmonary dysplasia in 34% headbox oxygen has an oxygen saturation of 100%.The partial pressure of oxygen is:
   a. 10 kPa
   b. 13.6 kPa
   c. 100 kPa
   d. cannot be determined from this information.

21.3 Concerning arterial blood gases:
   a. a normal pulse oximetry reading indicates normal blood gases
   b. the relation between pulse oximetry readings and arterial Po_2 is linear
   c. the arterial Po_2 may be normal in carbon monoxide poisoning
   d. the normal umbilical venous Po_2 is around 10 kPa in the fetus.

1.1 Wilms' tumour and neuroblastoma

1.2 Wilms' tumour – renal ischaemia; neuroblastoma – increased catecholamines secretions.

1.3 Wilms' tumour – lungs; neuroblastoma – long bones.

Discussion
Large unilateral abdominal masses arising from the renal angle strongly suggest a primary renal tumour (Wilms') or a neuroblastoma, although the asymptomatic nature of the presentation points more to a Wilms' tumour than neuroblastoma. Acquired hydronephrosis is also possible but one might have expected a history of urinary tract infections. Less likely is a congenitally large and abnormal kidney – most tend to be bilateral and present earlier.

Hypertension is more commonly present in Wilms' tumour than neuroblastoma. In Wilms', renal ischaemia is the main cause of hypertension, whereas in neuroblastoma circulating catecholamines secreted by the abnormal adrenal tissue lead to hypertension. Metastases in Wilms' tend to be confined to the lung. By contrast, neuroblastoma is often disseminated locally and remotely at presentation to long bones, the spinal column and liver.

| STATION 2 | ANSWERS | EXAM E |

2.1 A Reduced calcification (osteopenia) of the bones; splaying and cupping of the heads of the radius and ulnar.
Diagnosis: rickets.

B Generalized bone hyperdensity.
Diagnosis: osteopetrosis (marble bone disease).

C The femoral head is flattened, fragmented and shows sclerotic changes.
Diagnosis: Perthe's disease.

| STATION 3 | ANSWERS | EXAM E |

3.1 Muscle weakness.

3.2 Gower's sign.

3.3 Duchenne muscular dystrophy, raised creatinine phosphokinase (CPK).

3.4 Genetic counselling.

Discussion
John has delayed motor development, muscle weakness and learning difficulties. The manner in which he gets up to stand (Gower's sign) and the waddle gait indicate proximal muscle weakness.

The diagnosis of Duchenne's muscular dystrophy (DMD) involves finding of a raised creatinine phosphokinase and typical muscle biopsy findings. DNA probes looking for deletion of dystrophin gene loci on the X chromosome are also now possible. John's mother is pregnant and the developing fetus may be affected. It is imperative that his parents should receive genetic counselling as soon as possible. Prenatal sexing and DNA probing are possible to exclude an affected fetus and should be considered following genetic counselling.

DMD is an X-linked disorder with an incidence of 1 in 3500. Approximately one-third of cases are due to new mutations. The recurrence risk where there is a family history of the disease is 50% and where there is no history (as in this case) and normal maternal CPK approximately 10%. Initially children with DMD have subtle abnormalities in motor development and muscle weakness. The delayed development becomes increasingly obvious and weakness is progressive. Affected children are characterized by delayed walking (nearly all unaffected children are walking by 18 months and boys especially should be investigated where there is a delay) and are wheelchair bound by the age of 12 years. Many have learning difficulties and this is not an uncommon mode of referral even before the motor abnormalities are identified. Management is based upon maintaining mobility with physiotherapy and callipers.

| STATION 4 | ANSWERS | EXAM E |

4.1   Croup.

4.2   Parainfluenza A virus.

4.3   None of these.

4.4   a or b

Discussion
Most cases of stridor associated with an infective illness in this age group are likely to be due to acute laryngotracheobronchitis (croup). The usual aetiology of croup is the parainfluenza A virus. The diagnosis is based upon clinical findings only, i.e. no investigations are required. Viewing of the upper airway or taking a throat swab are particularly contraindicated as sudden severe laryngospasm may occur. The main differential diagnosis, acute epiglottitis, characterized by a 'toxic appearance', muffled voice and drooling in an older child, is now rare as a result of effective haemophilus influenza B immunization in infancy. Management involves rest in a comfortable environment with oxygen saturation monitoring. There is no evidence to support the use of humidity inside an oxygen tent. Antibiotics are not indicated. Nebulized budesonide and oral dexamethasone have been shown to attenuate the severity of the illness.

OSCEs in PAEDIATRICS

5.1 A purpuric skin rash.

5.2 Urticarial type skin lesions.

5.3 Henoch–Schönlein purpura.

5.4 Chronic glomerulonephritis leading to renal failure.

5.5 Blood pressure.

Discussion

Henoch–Schönlein purpura is the most common vasculitis syndrome affecting children. The small vessels of the skin, joints and viscera may all be affected. The skin manifestations include erythematous and urticarial type lesions but a purpuric rash principally affecting extensor surfaces, especially the buttocks and both legs, is characteristic. Arthritis with marked joint pain and swelling is usually self limiting and non-progressive. Colicky abdominal pain is also common; rarer is bowel perforation or intussusception. Renal involvement is usually not clinically apparent but can be inferred from urinalysis showing red and white cells and proteinuria. Abnormal urea and electrolytes or hypertension suggest more extensive renal involvement.

6.1 Intussusception.

6.2 Blood or bloody mucus.

6.3 a or b.

6.4 Peritonitis/intestinal perforation.

6.5 Fluid replacement followed by an open reduction via laporotomy.

Discussion

Intussusception is the invagination of a portion of intestine into itself. It occurs most commonly at the ileo-caecal valve, although no cause is usually found. The presentation is that of a well infant who suddenly develops vomiting and apparent colicky abdominal pain. Crying and drawing up the thighs with or without episodes of pallor and sweating occur. In between episodes the infant appears to recover, and is even playful. However, the episodes recur with shorter periods of well-being in between. Vomiting may become bile stained. There may be diarrhoea and significant dehydration may occur. Bloody mucus, often described as 'redcurrant' jelly stool may be passed in the nappy or noted on rectal examination. A sausage-shaped mass can be palpable in most cases.

A plain abdominal film or ulrasound will usually demonstrate the intussusception. A contrast Gastrograffin enema can also be used to reduce it. U&E must be monitored as dehydration and electrolyte imbalances occur frequently.

If there are signs of peritonitis, then an open reduction via a laporotomy must be carried out after circulatory failure has been corrected with intravenous fluid therapy.

| STATION 7 | ANSWERS | EXAM E |

7.1 false. This is the definition for perinatal mortality. Neonatal mortality is the number of deaths per 1000 live births during the first 28 days of life.

7.2 true

7.3 false

7.4 false

7.5 true

Discussion

Perinatal mortality more accurately reflects fetomaternal health and healthcare, whereas neonatal mortality reflects both this and neonatal healthcare – such as intensive care. Changes in maternal health such as increased numbers of teenage pregnancies are likely to be reflected by changes in perinatal mortality, whereas changes in infant care practices such as the use of surfactant are likely to be reflected in neonatal mortality rates.

It is probably true to say that the incidence of surfactant deficiency is on the decline because of the increasing use of steroids in threatened preterm labour, but this graph only shows a decrease in death from respiratory distress syndrome.

| STATION 8 | ANSWERS | EXAM E |

8.1 Volumatic – 3 years.

8.2 Babyhaler – 12 months.

8.3 Turbohaler – 8 years.

8.4 Metered dose inhaler – 15 years.

Discussion

An understanding of the principles of the most commonly used devices for delivering anti-asthma inhalation therapy is important for the delivery of anti-asthma care. Most children under the age of 4–5 years will not be able to coordinate inhalation with manual activation of the standard metered dose inhaler (MDI) or take a deep enough inhalation regularly to use a powdered

OSCEs IN PAEDIATRICS

dose inhaler. The most effective therapy, out of those given, is therefore a spacer device with an attached MDI plus or minus a facemask. The smaller volume spacers, e.g. Aerochamber and Babyhaler, are more suitable in infancy as their holding volume matches the tidal volume of this age group. Volumatic and nebuhaler devices in virtue of their larger volumes are, in general, more suitable for the 2 year and above age group. From age 7 years upwards, children tolerate powdered dose inhalers better. Clearly, some children prefer to use the device they are accustomed to and will be reluctant to change to a new one. On the whole, however, given sufficient explanation and practice coupled with the knowledge of convenience of carrying the device most children will prefer to use one of these, e.g. Accuhaler, Diskhaler or Turbohaler (as in this case). From teens upwards the standard MDI, although often well used, frequently causes difficulty in coordinating inhalation to actuation. This can be overcome by training or the use of a breath-actuated MDI, e.g. Autohaler.

| **STATION 9** | ANSWERS | **EXAM E** |

9.1 A. Cavernous haemangioma (strawberry naevus).
B. An extensive capillary haemangioma (associated in this case with Sturge–Weber syndrome). A scald would also be acceptable.
C. Haemorrhagic varicella (chickenpox).

| **STATION 10** | ANSWERS | **EXAM E** |

10.1 Hypochloraemic, hyponatraemic, hypokalaemic alkalosis.

10.2 Urinary tract infection, gastro-oesophageal reflux and congenital hypertrophic pyloric stenosis.

10.3 Congenital hypertrophic pyloric stenosis.

10.4 a, d and e.

Discussion
Congenital hypertrophic pyloric stenosis is more common in males and firstborns. There may also be a positive family history. The vomiting is projectile and not bile stained. The relation between vomiting and feeds can be variable but episodes of vomiting usually occur within half an hour of a feed and the infant is characteristically hungry afterwards. On examination infants are between 5 and 10% dehydrated. Gastric peristalsis may be visible. The 'pyloric tumour' is palpable during a test feed, especially after a vomit. Biochemical abnormalities reflect dehydration, loss of gastric secretions and secondary hyperaldosteronism; hyponatraemia, hypokalaemia, hypochloraemia and alkalosis. An abdominal ultrasound can be used to visualize the hypertrophied pylorus. UTI and gastro-oesophageal reflux need to be considered in the differential diagnoses. Urine should therefore always be checked for microscopy and culture. An increased white cell count would be consistent with a diagnosis of a UTI.

The treatment of congenital hypertrophic pyloric stenosis begins with correction of dehydration and electrolyte abnormalities with intravenous fluids and nasogastric drainage, followed by surgical repair.

STATION 11   ANSWERS   **EXAM E**

11.1   Autosomal recessive.

11.2   Cystic fibrosis and sickle cell disease.

11.3   The risk of 'A' being a carrier is 2/3.

11.4   The risk of 'A' having an affected child is 1/240.

Discussion

The most likely pattern of inheritance is autosomal recessive. These type of disorders are commonly severe and many of the inborn errors of metabolism are of this type. Other examples include thalassaemia, congenital adrenal hyperplasia and phenylketonuria.

On average one-quarter of children of carrier parents will be homozygous and normal, one-half heterozygous and phenotypically normal, and one-quarter homozygous and affected. The risk of 'A' being a carrier is therefore 2 out of 3. The risk of 'A' having affected children is 2/3 × 1/40 (this gives the chances of these two meeting), multiplied by the risk of having affected children, i.e. 1/4. This equals 2/3 × 1/40 × 1/4 = 1/240. Clearly if he has a consanguineous (commoner in Asian and Middle Eastern families) marriage the risk is increased.

STATION 12   ANSWERS   **EXAM E**

12.1   c

12.2   c

12.3   a

12.4   a

Discussion

This child has DiGeorge syndrome, a diagnosis which you would not be expected to identify. However, the fact that he is obviously 'syndromic' should alert you to the possibility that he may have abnormalities of internal structures and organs.

Left to right shunting of blood across a large ventricular septal defect increases the blood flow through the left atrium and across the mitral valve. Large shunts will manifest as diastolic murmurs because of increased flow across the mitral valve.

This child has no evidence of significant fluid overload (normal sodium) and venesection normally increases plasma calcium levels. With significant malabsorption one might expect a low albumin – the poor weight gain is

     OSCEs IN PAEDIATRICS

typical of infants with large ventricular septal defects. Congenital absence of the parathyroid gland causing primary hypoparathyroidism is the only likely explanation for the low calcium. This should make you suspect that other organs might be absent. The thymus gland is essential in programming developmental aspects of cell-mediated immunity. Its absence would predispose to fungal infections. Both the thymus and parathyroid glands develop from the 3rd and 4th pharyngeal pouches.

| STATION 13 | ANSWERS | EXAM E |

13.1 The right upper lobe is homogeneously hyperdense with loss of the cardiac border on the right upper side and an adjacent air bronchogram.

13.2 Right upper lobe pneumonia.

13.3 Analgesia and physiotherapy.

13.4 b

13.5 Repeat chest X-ray in approximately 4–8 weeks.

Discussion
This X-ray illustrates right upper lobe consolidation. The right cardiac silhouette is indistinct and there is an adjacent air bronchogram. The most likely underlying cause is a right upper lobe pneumonia. *Strep. pneumoniae* is the commonest cause of lobar pneumonia in the UK; the most appropriate antibiotic in this case is therefore penicillin. The intravenous form of this and, consequently, intravenous fluids would only be required if the child was systemically unwell or if oral intake was compromised. Resistance to penicillin is, however, increasing, and it may be that in a few years time a different antibiotic would be required. Analgesia/antipyretic and physiotherapy would be required. A 5–7-day course of antibiotic is normally given and the child brought back for a repeat chest X-ray in approximately 4–8 weeks time to ensure complete resolution of radiological signs has taken place. Significant persisting changes may require further investigation; e.g. bronchoscopy to exclude foreign body or search for other pathogens.

| STATION 14 | ANSWERS | EXAM E |

14.1 The following would indicate 'simple' bedwetting:
- a normal pattern of micturition, i.e. absence of dribbling/hesitation and strong urinary stream
- occasional dry nights
- a family history of bedwetting (which resolved) in a first degree relative
- normal development
- no polyuria or polydipsia
- absence of haematuria, dysuria and frequency.

OSCEs IN PAEDIATRICS

14.2 The urine should be tested for protein, blood, glucose and specific gravity. A clean specimen of urine should be sent for microscopy and culture to exclude infection.

14.3 c

Discussion

Bedwetting is a common problem and can affect children well into their teenage years. Simple questions and tests as outlined above should exclude secondary causes of bedwetting (e.g. UTI). Thereafter understanding, reassurance and patience are the mainstay of management. Simple measures such as not drinking too close to bedtime, voiding before bedtime and once again late at night are useful self-help measures. The success rates of bedwetting alarms are very variable. Intranasal DDAVP (a synthetic vasopressin analogue) spray will often stop bedwetting, but relapse is common and at present it is only used for short periods, e.g. the child is on holiday or during school examinations.

| **STATION 15** | ANSWERS | **EXAM E** |

15.1 See Discussion.

15.2 See Discussion.

15.3 *Neisseria meningitidis.*

15.4 a or c

15.5 rifampicin or ciprofloxacin.

Discussion

In bacterial meningitis, the CSF may have the following features:

- raised protein
- reduced CSF/blood glucose ratio
- raised white cell count
- turbidity – least useful or reliable.

During a 'bloody tap' cells from the blood enter the CSF. Under these circumstances a total white cell count can be misleading and a high white cell:red cell ratio (greater than 1 to 500) is used to indicate a significantly raised white cell count in the CSF. The presence of any pathogen on microscopy confirms the diagnosis. *Neisseria meningitides* is the causative organism in this case. Other causes of bacterial meningitis in the paediatric population are *Strep. pneumoniae* (Gram-positive cocci) and *Haemophilus influenzae* (Gram-negative bacilli). Treatment is with high-dose intravenous antibiotics – in this case benzylpenicillin or ceftriaxone is satisfactory. In situations where the microscopic diagnosis is not immediately available or is negative, third-generation cephalosporins – ceftriaxone or cefotaxime – must be given at least until culture results become available.

Nasopharyngeal carriage of the meningococcus in the host and in all household or close contacts requires treatment – in this case oral rifampicin is satisfactory. Ciprofloxacin can also be used.

OSCEs IN PAEDIATRICS

16.1, 16.2	Sitting up without support	8 months
	Pincer grip	9 months
	Walking	13 months
	Climbing stairs	15 months
16.3	11–15 months	
16.4	2–3 double syllable words with meaning, e.g. 'mama' and 'dada' to parents.	

Discussion
The ability to perform a development assessment is specific, as well as essential, to paediatric practice. Common milestones should be learnt. Some other examples are:

6 weeks	smiling, follows face in 90° arc, still's to mother's voice
4 months	rolls over front to back
6 months	palmar grasp, sits up with support, turns to voice
7–9 months	pulls self to stand
18 months	puts two words together, kicks ball, spoon feeds self

17.1 Throat swab, ASOT, cardiac echo, antinuclear factor, slit lamp examination of eyes looking for iritis, rheumatoid factor.

17.2 Rheumatic fever.

Discussion
Fiona has an asymmetrical developing arthropathy, a pyrexia of unknown origin (fever > 5 days) and possible cardiac involvement. The differential diagnosis includes rheumatic fever (poststreptococcal infection), juvenile chronic arthritis and systemic lupus erythematosus. The key features suggesting rheumatic fever in this case are preceding throat infection, presence of murmur and migratory arthritis. Other commonly associated features include erythema marginatum, subcutaneous nodules and the development of chorea. Investigations, not mentioned above, that would help confirm the diagnosis include ECG (to look for prolonged PR interval) and measurement of anti-DNAase and antihyaluronidase. Chest X-ray looking for cardiomegaly would also be acceptable.

18.1 The blood film shows atypical mononuclear cells which are enlarged with irregular nuclei and basophilic pleomorphic cytoplasm. The palate shows petechiae.

18.2 Infectious mononucleosis.

18.3 Thrombocytopenia, pneumonitis and splenic infarct.

18.4 Amoxycillin.

Discussion

The blood film showing atypical mononuclear cells and the palate showing petechiae are characteristic of infectious mononucleosis due to Epstein–Barr virus. Although this is usually a benign illness, severe multisystem complications are recognized. A debilitating meningoencephalitis may occur, confirmed by the presence of viral indices on CSF investigation. Hepatitis and thrombocytopenia are usually self-limiting. Pneumonitis can be serious and mortality has been associated with splenic inflammation and rupture. A severe tonsillopharyngitis can rarely compromise breathing. Amoxycillin and ampicillin should both be avoided as a florid maculopapular rash may occur.

STATION 19	ANSWERS	EXAM E

19.1

Age	Vaccine/s
2 months	Diphtheria, tetanus, pertussis, haem influen B and polio
3 months	Diphtheria, tetanus, pertussis, haem influen B and polio
4 months	Diphtheria, tetanus, pertussis, haem influen B and polio
12–18 months	Measles, mumps and rubella (MMR)
4–5 years	Diphtheria, tetanus, polio and MMR
10–14 years	BCG
15–18 years	Diphtheria, tetanus and polio

Note: BCG and hepatitis B are offered to those at risk at birth.

STATION 20	ANSWERS	EXAM E

20.1 220 beats/min.

20.2 Supraventricular tachycardia (SVT).

20.3 Sudden dipping of her face in *ice cold* water. Applying ocular pressure is not recommended. A parasympathetic (vagal) response is elicited which has a negative chronotropic effect.

Discussion

An SVT is characterized by a rapid heart rate (>200–280 beats/min), normal looking QRS complexes and P waves that are difficult to identify in the rhythm strip because at these very fast rates they are 'buried' in the T wave of the preceding QRS complex. SVTs generally occur in structurally normal hearts and may be secondary to thyrotoxicosis and coxsackie infection. The most common association is with Wolff–Parkinson–White syndrome which is due to an anomalous conduction pathway between the atria and ventricles (bundle of Kent).

STATION 21	ANSWERS	EXAM E

21.1 a

21.2 d

21.3 c – true; the rest are false.

Discussion

Pulse oximeters are in widespread use and it is important to know their use and limitations. These questions test your understanding of the oxyhaemoglobin dissociation curve.

Pulse oximeters measure the percentage of haemoglobin which is oxygenated. At 100% saturation the oximetry reading is on the 'flat' part of the oxyhaemoglobin dissociation curve and so it is impossible to know the partial pressure of oxygen. A pulse oximeter does not measure carbon dioxide or pH and gives no information about CO_2 retention or acid–base status. The oxyhaemoglobin dissociation curve is sigmoid and so is the relation between pulse oximetry readings and arterial Po_2.

Arterial blood gas machines measure the partial pressure of oxygen dissolved in whole blood and not the amount of oxygen bound to haemoglobin. Hence in CO poisoning which binds to haemoglobin 20 times more effectively than oxygen the Po_2 may be normal.

The fetal Po_2 varies slightly with gestation but most studies show it to be between 2.5 and 4.5 kPa.